MCA

Rules and Guidance for Pharmaceutical Manufacturers 1993

incorporating:

- EC Guide to GMP
- EC Directives on GMP
- Code of Practice for Qualified Persons
- Standard Provisions for Manufacturer's Licences

LONDON: HMSO

First published 1993

ISBN 0 11 321633 5

CONTENTS

Introduction 3

Acknowledgements 4

Part 1 Standard Provisions for Manufacturer's and Wholesale Dealer's (Import) Licences; Prescribed Conditions for Manufacturer's Undertakings for Imported Products 5

Part 2 Code of Practice for Qualified Persons 19

Part 3 The GMP Directives 91/356/EEC and 91/341/EEC 29

Part 4 Guide to GMP for Medicinal Products 39

Annexes 89

Glossary 169

Index 177

Part 5 Defective Medicines Report Centre 193

INTRODUCTION

This publication brings together the main pharmaceutical regulations, directives and guidance which a manufacturer is expected to follow when making medicinal products. It is of particular relevance to all holders of Manufacturer's Licences and to their Qualified Persons who have a responsibility for ensuring compliance with many of these requirements.

The obligation on governments of all Member States of the European Community to ensure that pharmaceutical manufacturers are authorised is stated in Chapter IV of Directive 75/319/EEC (products for human use) and Chapter V of Directive 81/851/EEC (veterinary products). These Chapters are also the source of requirements for compliance with Good Manufacturing Practice (GMP), employment of Qualified Persons and repeated inspections by the regulatory authorities.

The Principles and Guidelines of GMP are stated in the two almost identical Directives, 91/356/EEC for medicinal products for human use and 91/341/EEC for veterinary medicinal products. In the United Kingdom the Directives have been implemented by standard provisions and undertakings incorporated in regulations made under the Medicines Act. Whereas before 1992 there was no specific legal requirement to comply with GMP, compliance with the principles and guidelines of GMP is now a statutory requirement. The European Community Guide to GMP provides detailed guidance which interprets and expands on the statutory Principles and Guidelines.

The UK first produced a national guide to GMP (known affectionately as the "Orange Guide" from the colour of its cover) in 1971. Two further editions were produced in 1977 and 1983. The EC Guide, issued first in 1989 and reprinted with minor corrections and additional annexes in 1992, supercedes this and all other national guides of Member States, although much that was familiar in the old UK Guide can be recognised in the EC Guide. Further annexes (numbers 13 and 14) were adopted in 1993. The Pharmaceutical Inspection Convention has also adopted the text of the EC Guide ensuring harmonisation of guidelines throughout Europe and beyond.

Manufacturers are required to name a Qualified Person on their Manufacturer's Licence. No batch of medicinal product may be released to the market within the EC unless a nominated Qualified Person has certified that it has been manufactured and checked in compliance with the laws in force. Guidance to Qualified Persons in fulfilling their responsibilities is given in the Code of Practice for Qualified Persons.

The object of good manufacturing practice and associated rules and guidelines is the assurance of the quality of the product for the safety, well-being and protection of the patient. In achieving this aim it is impossible to over-emphasise the importance of people, at all levels, in the assurance of the quality of medicinal products. This is emphasised in the first principle in the Guide to GMP. The great majority of reported defective medicinal products has resulted from human error or carelessness, not from failures in technology. All the people involved with the production, quality control or distribution of medicinal products, whether key personnel, production or control staff, medicines inspectors or others involved in the many activities which lead to a patient taking a medicine, should bear this constantly in mind when performing their duties.

ACKNOWLEDGEMENTS

To the European Commission for permission to reproduce the text of the Directives and Guide to GMP.

To the Institute of Biology, the Royal Pharmaceutical Society of Great Britain and the Royal Society of Chemistry for permission to use the text of the Code of Practice for Qualified Persons.

Part One

Standard provisions for manufacturer's and wholesale dealer's (import) licences

Prescribed conditions for manufacturer's undertakings for imported products

1 STANDARD PROVISIONS FOR LICENCES

Extracts from

The Medicines (Standard Provisions for Licences and Certificates) Regulations 1971 (SI 1971 No 972) as amended by Amendment Regulations 1972 (SI 1972 No 1226), 1977 (SI 1977 No 1053). 1983 (SI 1983 No. 1730) and 1992 (SI 1992 No. 2846)

Note

These extracts from the Regulations are presented for the reader's convenience and incorporate amendments up to the end of 1992. For any definitive information reference must be made to the original Regulations. ***Also for convenience, the amendments introduced in 1992 in order to comply with Directive 91/356/EEC are reproduced in italics; this device has no statutory significance.***

Interpretation

[The following definitions of terms used in the Standard Provisions for Manufacturer's Licences are inserted by SI 1992 No. 2846 to Regulation 2.1 of the Principal Regulations:]

"expiry date", in relation to a medicinal product, means the date after which the product should not be used.

"good manufacturing practice" means the part of quality assurance which ensures that medicinal products are consistently produced and controlled to the quality standards appropriate to their intended use, the principles and guidelines of which are specified in Chapter II of Commission Directive 91/356/EEC.

"relevant period" means the period of five years from the date of certification of the relevant batch referred to in paragraph 16(3)(b) of Schedule 2 to these Regulations or the period of one year from the expiry date of the relevant batch, whichever expires later.

Schedule 2 of the Regulations: Standard Provisions For Manufacturer's Licences

1. The licence holder shall provide and maintain such staff, premises and plant as are necessary for the carrying out in accordance with his licence and the relevant product licences of such stages of the manufacture and assembly of the medicinal prod-

ucts as are undertaken by him, and he shall not carry out any such manufacture or assembly except at the premises specified in his manufacturer's licence.

2. The licence holder shall provide and maintain such staff, premises, equipment and facilities for the handling, storage and distribution of the medicinal products which he handles, stores or distributes under his licence as are necessary to avoid deterioration of the medicinal products and he shall not use for such purposes premises other than those specified in the licence or which may be approved from time to time by the licensing authority.

3. The licence holder shall conduct all manufacture and assembly operations in such a way as to ensure that the medicinal products conform with the standards of strength, quality and purity applicable to them under the relevant product licences *and, in relation to medicinal products for human use, shall conduct all such operations in accordance with the principles and guidelines of good manufacturing practice*

3A. The licence holder shall, in relation to medicinal products for human use, establish and implement an effective pharmaceutical quality assurance system involving the active participation of the management and personnel of the different services involved.

4. The licence holder, where animals are used in the production of any medicinal products and the relevant product licences contain provisions relating to them, shall arrange for the animals to be housed in premises of such a nature and to be managed in such a way as will facilitate compliance with such provisions.

5. The licence holder shall, *in relation to medicinal products, other than for human use,* either

   (a) provide and maintain such staff, premises and plant as are necessary for carrying out in accordance with the relevant product licences any tests of the strength, quality and purity of the medicinal products that he manufactures under his manufacturer's licence as required by those product licences, and when animals are used for such tests they shall be suitably housed and managed, or

   (b) make arrangements with a person approved by the licensing authority for such tests to be carried out in accordance with the relevant product licences on his behalf by that person.

5A (1) The licence holder shall, in relation to medicinal products for human use –

   (a) provide and maintain a designated quality control department having authority in relation to quality control and being independent from all other departments in the exercise of that authority; and

   (b) place the quality control department under the authority of the person notified to the licensing authority in accordance with paragraph 7(2) of Schedule 1 to the Medicines (Applications for Manufacturer's and Wholesale Dealer's Licences) Regulations 1971(SI 1971/974) as being responsible for quality control.

(2) Subject to paragraph 5B of this Schedule, the licence holder shall, in order to support the quality control department, provide and maintain such staff, premises and plant as are necessary for carrying out –

(a) such tests of the strength, quality and purity of the medicinal products which he manufactures for human use under the manufacturer's licence as are required by the relevant product licences, and

(b) any tests or controls which relate to the conditions of production and in-process controls.

(3) Any animals used for the tests referred to in sub-paragraph (2) of this paragraph shall be suitably housed and managed.

(4) The licence holder shall ensure that the quality control department, in determining whether finished medicinal products for human use are to be released for sale or distribution, takes into account, in addition to analytical results –

(a) the conditions of production,

(b) the result of in-process controls,

(c) the examination of manufacturing documents, and

(d) the conformity of products to the specification in the relevant product licence.

5B. A licence holder need not himself provide and maintain such staff, premises and plant as are necessary for carrying out such tests as are specified in paragraph 5A(2) of this Schedule provided that he makes arrangements with a person approved by the licensing authority to carry out such tests on his behalf in accordance with paragraph 5A(2) and (3) of this Schedule.

6. The licence holder shall provide such information as may be requested by the licensing authority for the purposes of the Act, about the products currently being manufactured or assembled under his licence and of the operations being carried out in relation to such manufacture or assembly.

7. The licence holder shall inform the licensing authority before making any material alteration in the premises or plant used under his licence, or in the operations for which they are used, and he shall inform the licensing authority of any change that he proposes to make in any personnel named in his licence as respectively:

(a) responsible for supervising the production operations, or

(b) responsible for quality control of the medicinal products being manufactured or assembled, including the person named as the qualified person for the purposes of paragraph 16 or l7, as the case may be, of this Part of this Schedule, or

(c) in charge of the animals from which are derived any substances used in the production of the medicinal products being manufactured or assembled, or

(d) responsible for the culture of any living tissues used in the manufacture of the medicinal products being manufactured or assembled.

8. The licence holder shall keep readily available for inspection by a person authorised by the licensing authority durable records of the details of manufacture and assembly of each batch of every medicinal product being manufactured or assembled under his licence and of the tests carried out thereon, including any register or other record referred to in paragraph 16(3)(b), or 17(3)(b), as the case may be, in such a form that the records will be easily identifiable from the number of the batch as shown on each container in which the medicinal product is sold, supplied or exported, and he shall permit the person authorised to take copies or make extracts from such records. Such records shall not be destroyed without the consent of the licensing authority

   (a) in relation to a medicinal product for human use, for the relevant period,

   (b) in any other case, for a period of five years from the date when the manufacture or assembly of the relevant batch occurred.

8A. The licence holder shall keep readily available for examination by a person authorised by the licensing authority samples of each batch of finished medicinal products for human use manufactured or assembled under his licence for at least a period of one year from their expiry date and shall retain samples of starting materials (other than solvents, gases or water) for at least a period of two years from the date of the release of the relevant batch of which the relevant starting materials formed part, except where the licence holder is authorised by the licensing authority to destroy any such samples earlier.

8B. The licence holder shall make suitable arrangements to ensure that any record or sample referred to in paragraphs 8 or 8A above relating to a medicinal product for human use is retained for the relevant period.

9. The licence holder shall, *in relation to medicinal products other than for human use,* keep such documents as will facilitate the withdrawal or recall from sale, supply or exportation of any such medicinal products to which the licence relates.

9A. (1) The licence holder shall implement a system for recording. and reviewing complaints in relation to medicinal products for human use manufactured or assembled under his licence, together with an effective system for recalling promptly and at any time such medicinal products in the distribution network.

(2) The licence holder shall record and investigate all complaints described in sub-paragraph (1) of this paragraph and shall immediately inform the licensing authority of any defect which could result in a recall from sale, supply or exportation or in an abnormal restriction on such sale, supply or exportation.

10. Where the licence holder has been informed by the licensing authority that any batch of any medicinal product to which his licence relates has been found not to conform as regards strength, quality or purity with the specification of the relevant product or with the provisions of the Act or of any regulations under the Act that are applicable to the medicinal product, he shall, if so directed, withhold such batch

from sale, supply or exportation, so far as may be reasonably practicable, for such a period not exceeding six weeks as may be specified by the licensing authority.

11. The licence holder shall ensure that any tests for determining conformity with the standards and specifications applying to any particular product used in the manufacture shall, except so far as the conditions of the relevant product licence may otherwise provide, be applied to samples from the medicinal product after all manufacturing processes have been completed, or at such earlier stage in the manufacture as may be approved by the licensing authority.

12. (1) The licence holder who is not the holder of a product licence in respect of the medicinal product to which the manufacturer's licence relates, shall comply with any provisions of such a product licence that relates to the sale of that medicinal product and shall, by means of a label or otherwise, communicate the particulars of such provisions as relate to mode of sale, or restriction as to sale, to any person to whom the licence holder sells or supplies that medicinal product.

(2) Where the manufacturer's licence relates to the assembly of a medicinal product, and the licence holder sells or supplies that medicinal product at such a stage of assembly that does not fully comply with the provisions of the relevant product licence that relates to labelling, that licence holder shall communicate the particulars of those provisions to the person to whom that medicinal product has been so sold or supplied.

13. Where in his application for a manufacturer's licence the licence holder had specified a general classification of medicinal products in respect of which that licence was required or had given particulars of manufacturing operations and of substances or articles in accordance with paragraph 6 of Schedule 1 to the Medicines (Applications for Manufacturer's and Wholesale Dealer's Licences) Regulations 1971 (SI 1971/974) and there has been, or it is proposed that there shall be, a change in such general classification or such particulars, the licence holder shall forthwith notify the licensing authority in writing of such change or proposed change.

14. Where the manufacturer's licence relates to the assembly of a medicinal product and that medicinal product is not manufactured by the licence holder, and where particulars as to the name and address of the manufacturer of, or of the person who imports, that medicinal product had been given by the licence holder to the licensing authority, the licence holder shall forthwith notify the licensing authority in writing of any changes in such particulars.

15. The licence holder, for the purpose of enabling the licensing authority to ascertain whether there are any grounds for suspending, revoking or varying any licence or certificate granted or issued under Part II of the Act, shall permit, and provide all necessary facilities to enable, any person duly authorised in writing by the licensing authority, on production if required of his credentials, to carry out such inspection or

to take such samples or copies, in relation to things belonging to, or any business carried on by, the licence holder, as such person would have the right to carry out or take under the Act for the purpose of verifying any statement contained in an application for a licence or certificate.

16 (1) Subject to sub-paragraph (5) below, the licence holder shall at all times have at his disposal the services of a person who as respects qualifications and experience satisfies the provisions of Articles 23 and 24 of the Second Council Directive, to carry out the functions specified in sub-paragraph (3) below ("qualified person"). For the purposes of this paragraph, but without prejudice to sub-paragraph (4) below, the licence holder may regard a person as satisfying the provisions of the said Article 24 as respects formal qualifications if he produces evidence that he is a member of the Pharmaceutical Society or of the Royal Institute of Chemistry or of such other body as may appear to the licensing authority to be an appropriate body for the purpose, and that he is regarded by the body of which he is a member as so satisfying those provisions.

(2) The licence holder shall at all times provide and maintain such staff, premises, equipment and facilities as will enable the qualified person who is at his disposal to carry out the said functions.

(3) The functions to be carried out by the qualified person shall be as follows:–

(a) To ensure that each batch of the medicinal product to which the licence relates has been manufactured or assembled and checked in compliance with the provisions of the Act and regulations made thereunder, the provisions of the licence and the provisions of the product licence which relates to the product;

(b) to certify in a register, or other record appropriate for the purpose, whether each production batch of the medicinal product to which the licence relates satisfies the requirements set out in (a) above and to ensure that such register or other record is regularly maintained, in particular that the appropriate entries in such register or other record are made as soon as practicable after each such batch has been manufactured.

(4) Where, after giving the licence holder and the person acting as a qualified person the opportunity of making representations to them (orally or in writing), the licensing authority are of the opinion that the person so acting does not satisfy the provisions of the said Articles 23 and 24 of the Second Council Directive as respects qualifications and experience, or that he is failing to carry out the functions specified in sub-paragraph (3) above, and have notified the licence holder accordingly in writing, the licence holder shall not permit that person to act as a qualified person so long as the said notification has not been withdrawn by the licensing authority.

(5) The provisions of this paragraph shall not apply in relation to veterinary drugs or to *[section deleted]* medicinal products that are homoeopathic products.

(6) The provisions of this paragraph shall also not apply where the licence relates to manufacturing activity which: –

(a) is limited to medicinal products to which Article 2 of the Medicines (Exemption from Licences) (Special and Transitional Cases) Order 1971 (SI 1971/1450) as amended (SI 1972/1200) applies, and consists solely of mixing together medicinal products and ingredients, other than active ingredients, on premises of which the licence holder is the occupier and which he is able to close so as to exclude the public, or

(b) is limited to assembly only, where all the products to be assembled are for sale or supply in the course of a business and are supplied, without any recommendation, for the purpose of administration to a particular person after the licence holder has been requested by or on behalf of that person, and in that person's presence, to use his judgement as to the treatment required.

(7) The provisions of this paragraph shall not have effect until 22nd November 1977 in relation to a licence which has been granted before the coming into operation of these regulations.

17\. (1) Subject to sub-paragraph (5) below, the licence holder shall at all times have at his disposal the services of a person who as respects qualifications and experience satisfies the provisions of Articles 31 and 32 of the Council Directive, to carry out the functions specified in sub-paragraph (3) below ("qualified person"). For the purposes of this paragraph, but without prejudice to sub-paragraph (4) below, the licence holder may regard a person as satisfying the provisions of the said Article 32 as respects formal qualifications if he produces evidence that he is a member of the Pharmaceutical Society or of the Royal Society of Chemistry or of such other body as may appear to the licensing authority to be an appropriate body for the purpose, and that he is regarded by the body of which he is a member as so satisfying those provisions.

(2) The licence holder shall at all times provide and maintain such staff, premises, equipment and facilities as will enable the qualified person who is at his disposal to carry out the said functions.

(3) The functions to be carried out by the qualified person shall be as follows:–

(a) to ensure that each batch of the medicinal product to which the licence relates has been manufactured or assembled and checked in compliance with the provisions of the Act and regulations made thereunder, the provisions of the licence and the provisions of the product licence which relates to the product;

(b) to certify in a register, or other record appropriate for the purpose, whether each production batch of the medicinal product to which the licence relates satisfies the requirements set out in (a) above and to ensure that such register or other record is regularly maintained, in particular that the appropriate entries in such register or other record are made as soon as practicable after each such batch has been manufactured.

(4) Where, after giving the licence holder and the person acting as a qualified person the opportunity of making representations to them (orally or in writing), the licensing authority are of the opinion that the person so acting does not satisfy the provisions of the said Articles 31 and 32 of the Council Directive as respects qualifications and experience, or that he is failing to carry out the functions specified in sub-paragraph (3) above, and have notified the licence holder accordingly in writing, the licence holder shall not permit that person to act as a qualified person so long as the said notification has not been withdrawn by the licensing authority.

(5) The provisions of this paragraph shall not apply in relation to:–

(a) medicinal products which are manufactured, sold, supplied, imported or exported for use by being administered to human beings.

(b) veterinary drugs which:–

(i) consist of vaccines, toxins or serums;

(ii) are based on radioactive isotopes;

(iii) are homoeopathic veterinary drugs; or

(iv) are additives for animal feeding stuffs to which the provisions of Council Directive 70/524/EEC apply.

(6) The provisions of this paragraph shall also not apply where the licence relates to manufacturing activity which:–

(a) is limited to medicinal products to which Article 2 of the Medicines (Exemptions from Licences) (Special and Transitional Cases) Order 1971 (SI 1971/1450 as amended by SI 1972/1200) applies, and consists solely of mixing together medicinal products and ingredients, other than active ingredients, on premises of which the licence holder is the occupier and which he is able to close so as to exclude the public; or

(b) is limited to assembly only, where all the products to be assembled are for sale or supply in the course of a business and are supplied, without any recommendation, for the purpose of administration to a particular animal or herd after the licence holder has been requested by the owner of that animal or herd to use his judgement as to the treatment required.

(7) The provisions of this paragraph shall not have effect until 9th October 1984 in relation to a licence which has been granted before the coming into operation of those regulations.

Schedule 3 of the Regulations: Standard Provisions For Wholesale Dealer's Licences

[The following paragraph is inserted by SI 1992 No. 2846 after paragraph 8 of Schedule 3 of the Principal Regulations]

"8A Where the licence relates to imported proprietary products, the licence holder shall in relation to medicinal products for human use –*

(a) ensure that all manufacture and assembly operations have been carried out by a duly authorised manufacturer or assembler and that the products have been manufactured and assembled in accordance with the principles and guidelines of good manufacturing practice;

(b) keep readily available for examination by a person authorised by the licensing authority samples of each batch of finished products for at least one year after their expiry date except where the licence holder is authorised by the licensing authority to destroy such samples earlier:

(c) implement a system for recording and reviewing complaints relating to the medicinal products to which his licence relates, together with an effective system for recalling promptly and at any time any such medicinal product in the distribution network; and

(d) record and investigate all such complaints and immediately inform the licensing authority of any defect which could result in a recall from sale, supply or exportation or in an abnormal restriction on such sale, supply or exportation."

2. PRESCRIBED CONDITIONS FOR MANUFACTURER'S UNDERTAKINGS FOR IMPORTED PRODUCTS

Extracts from

The Medicines (Manufacturer's Undertakings for Imported Products) Regulations 1977 (SI 1977 No 1038) as amended by Amendment Regulations 1992 (SI 1992 No 2845)

Note

This extract from the Regulations is presented for the reader's convenience. For any definitive information reference must be made to the original Regulations. ***Also for convenience, the amendments introduced in 1992 in order to comply with Directive 91/356/EEC are reproduced in italics; this device has no statutory significance.***

---

* "imported proprietary product" means a proprietary medicinal product imported other than from a member state. See: "interpretation" in SI 1971 No. 972.

[An additional regulation (regulation 4) is inserted by SI 1992 No. 2845 to exclude from the scope of the regulations applications for products coming from another member state of the EEC]

Schedule: Prescribed Conditions for Manufacturer's Undertakings

1. The manufacturer shall provide and maintain such staff, premises and plant as are necessary for the carrying out in accordance with the relevant product licences of such stages of the manufacture and assembly of the medicinal products to which the relevant product licences relate as are undertaken by him.

2. The manufacturer shall provide and maintain such staff, premises, equipment and facilities for the handling, storage and distribution of the medicinal products to which the relevant product licences relate which he handles, stores or distributes as are necessary to avoid deterioration of the medicinal products.

2A. In relation to medicinal products for human use, the manufacturer shall provide and maintain a designated quality control department having authority in relation to quality control and being independent of all other departments.

3. The manufacturer shall conduct all manufacture and assembly operations in such a way as to ensure that the medicinal products to which the relevant product licences relate conform with the standards of strength, quality and purity applicable to them under the relevant product licences.

3A. In relation to medicinal products for human use, the manufacturer shall maintain an effective pharmaceutical quality assurance system involving the active participation of the management and personnel of the different services involved.

4. Where animals are used in the production of any medicinal product and the relevant product licences contain provisions relating to them the manufacturer shall arrange for the animals to be housed in premises of such a nature and to be managed in such a way as will facilitate compliance with such provisions.

5. The manufacturer shall make such adequate and suitable arrangements as are necessary for carrying out in accordance with the relevant product licences any tests of the strength, quality or purity of the medicinal products to which the licences relate.

6. The manufacturer shall inform the holder of the relevant product licences of any material alteration in the premises or plant used in connection with the manufacture or assembly of the medicinal products to which the relevant product licences relate or in the operations for which such premises or plant are so used and of any change, since the granting of the relevant product licences in respect of any person:–
   (a) responsible for supervising the production operations, or
   (b) responsible for quality control of the medicinal products to which the relevant product licences relate, or

(c) in charge of the animals from which are derived any substance used in the production of the medicinal products to which the relevant product licences relate, or

(d) responsible for the culture of any living tissues used in the manufacture of the medicinal products to which the relevant product licences relate.

7. The manufacturer shall keep readily available for inspection by a person authorised by the licensing authority durable records of the details of manufacture and assembly of each batch of every medicinal product to which each relevant product licence relates and of the tests carried out thereon in such a form that the records will be easily identifiable from the number of the batch as shown on each container in which the medicinal product is exported from the country where it has been manufactured or assembled; the manufacturer shall permit the person authorised to take copies of or make extracts from such records. Such records shall not be destroyed –

(a) in relation to a medicinal product for human use, for a period of five years from the date of release of the relevant batch, or for a period of one year after the expiry date of the relevant batch, whichever expires later,

(b) in any other case.

7A. In relation to medicinal products for human use to which a product licence relates, the manufacturer shall keep readily available for examination by a person authorised by the licensing authority, samples of –

(a) each batch of finished products for at least a period of one year after their expiry date; and

(b) starting materials (other than solvents, gases or water) for at least a period of two years after release of the medicinal product of which the relevant starting materials formed part;

except where the manufacturer is authorised by the licensing authority to destroy such samples earlier.

7B (1) The manufacturer shall implement a system for recording and reviewing complaints in relation to medicinal products for human use to which a product licence relates together with an effective system for recalling promptly and at any time the medicinal products in the distribution network.

(2) The manufacturer shall record and investigate all complaints described in sub-paragraph (1) of this paragraph and shall immediately inform the licensing authority of any defect which could result in a recall from sale, supply or exportation or in an abnormal restriction on such sale, supply or exportation.

8. The manufacturer shall inform the holder of the relevant product licence of any material change since the date upon which such licence was granted in respect of: –

(a) the facilities and equipment available at each of the premises of the manufacturer for carrying out any stage of the manufacture or assembly of the medicinal products to which the relevant product licences relate, or

(b) the facilities and equipment available in each of the premises of the manufacturer for the storage of the medicinal products to which the relevant product licences relate on, and distribution of the products from or between, such premises, or

(c) any manufacturing operations, not being operations in relation to the medicinal products to which the relevant product licences relate, which are carried on by the manufacturer on or near any of the premises on which such medicinal products are manufactured or assembled and the substances or articles in respect of which such operations are carried on, or

(d) the arrangements for the identification and storage of materials and ingredients before and during manufacture of the medicinal products to which the relevant product licences relate and the arrangements for the storage of the medicinal products after they have been manufactured or assembled, or

(e) the arrangements for ensuring satisfactory turnover of stocks of medicinal products to which the relevant product licences relate, or

(f) the arrangements for maintaining production records and records of analytical and other testing procedures applied in the course of manufacture or assembly of the medicinal products to which the relevant product licences relate, or

(g) the arrangements for keeping reference samples of materials used in the manufacture of any medicinal products to which the relevant product licences relate and reference samples of such medicinal products.

Part Two

Code of practice for qualified persons

QUALIFIED PERSONS

Note

All holders of Manufacturer's Licences or Wholesale Dealer (Import) Licences are required to have available the services of a Qualified Person (QP), who must be named on their licence. When considering a nomination, the Licensing Authority routinely takes into account the assessment of the nominee's eligibility made either by the Institute of Biology, the Royal Pharmaceutical Society of Great Britain or the Royal Society of Chemistry, according to which body the person belongs. Exceptionally the Medicines Control Agency will assess a nominee directly if he or she is not a member of any of these professional bodies.

Chapter IV of Directive 75/319/EEC lays down the requirements for Qualified Persons in relation to products for human use. Article 22 defines the duties of the QP, Articles 23 and 24 define the requirements for eligibility under the permanent and transistional arrangements respectively, and Article 25 requires Member States to ensure that the duties of QPs are fulfilled, either through administrative measures or by making such persons subject to a professional code of conduct. Chapter V of Directive 81/851/EEC lays down equivalent requirements in relation to veterinary products.

By inspection and other means the Licensing Authority routinely assesses whether or not QPs are fulfilling their duties. In making this assessment, reference is made to the Code of Practice for Qualified Persons produced jointly by the Institute of Biology, the Royal Pharmaceutical Society of Great Britain and the Royal Society of Chemistry in collaboration with the Medicines Control Agency and the Veterinary Medicines Directorate. This reference is made whether or not the Qualified Person in question is a member of one or more of these bodies.

All Qualified Persons should be guided in fulfilling their duties by this Code of Practice, although the references in sections 9.1 and 10.4 to the disciplinary machinery of the professional bodies, and in section 9.5(b) to the advice which professional bodies can give, would not be relevant in the case of a Qualified Person who is not a member of one of these bodies.

The Medicines Control Agency acknowledges with thanks the Societies' permission to reproduce the Code below as revised in May 1993.

Code of Practice for Qualified Persons

1.0 Purpose of the Code

The legal functions of the Qualified Person (QP) are stated in SI 1971 No. 972 (as amended). The aims and objectives of this Code of Practice are to provide operational guidelines for carrying out these functions within a professional code of conduct in the interests of Qualified Persons, their employers, patients, the Medicines Control Agency (MCA) of the Department of Health and the Veterinary Medicines Directorate (VMD) of the Ministry of Agriculture, Fisheries and Foods. This code applies equally to human and veterinary medicines.

2.0 Application of the Code

The Code shall apply equally to Qualified Persons who have achieved that status under the transitional arrangements or the permanent provisions.

Qualified Persons have a professional duty to decline to act as QPs for release of product types for which they do not possess the relevant experience and knowledge; this may apply especially to those who achieve that status under the transitional arrangements.

3.0 Terminology

The terminology used in this Code of Practice corresponds with that used in the European Community Guide to Good Manufacturing Practice for Medicinal Products 1992.

In the Guide to GMP 1992 the terms Marketing Authorisation and Manufacturing Authorisation are equivalent to Product Licence (PL) and Manufacturer's Licence (ML) issued under the UK licensing system, and shall henceforth be referred to throughout this Code as PL and ML.

4.0 General Principles for the Manufacture of medicinal Products

Pharmaceutical Manufacturers and the Licensing Authorities have a duty to assure the general public that patients are properly protected and that medicinal products meet appropriate requirements for safety, quality and efficacy. The legal framework is provided by the European Directives and Rules governing medicinal products, United Kingdom primary legislation notably the Medicines Act 1968, and by subsequent statutory instruments.

Operational guidelines are provided in Volume IV of the Rules – the EC Guide to GMP for Medicinal Products. In Chapter 1 of the Guide, Quality Management, it states that:

> "The holder of a Manufacturing Authorisation must manufacture medicinal products so as to ensure that they are fit for their intended use, comply with the requirements of the Marketing Authorisation and do not place patients at risk due to inadequate safety, quality or efficacy. The attainment of this quality objective is the responsibility of senior management and requires the participation and commitment by staff in many different departments and at all levels within the company, the company's suppliers and the distributors.

To achieve the quality objective reliably there must be a comprehensively designed and correctly implemented system of Quality Assurance incorporating Good Manufacturing Practice and thus Quality Control. It should be fully documented and its effectiveness monitored. All parts of the Quality Assurance system should be adequately resourced with competent personnel, and suitable and sufficient premises, equipment and facilities. There are additional legal responsibilities for the holder of the Manufacturing Authorisation and for the Qualified Person(s).

The basic concepts of Quality Assurance, Good Manufacturing Practice and Quality Control are inter-related. They are described here in order to emphasise their relationships and their fundamental importance to the production and control of medicinal products".

Quality Management extends to original product design, development, formulation and preparation of medicinal products for use in clinical trials. This includes the establishment of well-defined manufacturing processes, sampling programmes and analytical test methods and appropriate specifications for ingredients, printed and unprinted packaging components and finished dosage forms.

Subsequently any pharmaceutical preparation should contain the same or a lesser range of impurities as the batch(es) used in clinical trials. It is therefore of vital importance that the quality of routine production batches should correspond to a specification derived from the composition of development batches. Ultimately the quality and safety of a medicinal product depends on the application of appropriate procedures based on GMP leading to a product within the recognised specification. Standard procedures and recognised specifications cannot be divorced.

5.0 Routine Duties of a Qualified Person

Qualified Persons have duties, some of which may be delegated (see later), in line with the above General Principles. Before certifying a batch prior to release the QP doing so should always ensure that the following requirements have been met:

5.1 The Product (PL) and the Manufacturer's Licence (ML) requirements for the medicinal product have been met for the batch concerned.

5.2 The principles and guidelines of good manufacturing practice as laid down in Directive 91/356/EEC (Human) or Directive 91/412/EEC (Veterinary) and interpreted in the "EC Guide to GMP" have been followed.

5.3 The principal manufacturing and testing processes have been validated.

5.4 All the necessary checks and tests have been performed and account taken of the production conditions and manufacturing records.

5.5 Any planned changes or deviations in manufacturing or quality control have been notified in accordance with a well defined reporting system before any product is released. Such changes may need notification to and approval by the MCA.

5.6 Any additional sampling, inspection, tests and checks have been carried out or initiated, as approprate, to cover planned changes or deviations.

5.7 All necessary production and QC documentation has been completed and endorsed by supervisors, trained in appropriate disciplines.

5.8 Appropriate audits, self-inspections and spot checks are being carried out by experienced staff.

5.9 All relevant factors have been considered including any not specifically associated with the output batch directly under review (e.g. sub-division of output batches from a common input, factors associated with continuous production runs).

5.10 The legal requirements regarding imported products have been fully met;

In considering these points the Qualified Person should recognise the need to consult her or his company's technical experts in the various areas of the Study Guide to reinforce the knowledge on appropriate points when a doubtful situation arises (e.g. increased levels of impurity, new impurities, plant/microbiological factors, etc).

6.0 Number and Location of Qualified Persons

The provisions of Statutory Instrument 1977, No. 1053 (Human Medicines) and Statutory Instrument 1983, No. 1730 (Veterinary Medicines) and the principles outlined in the EC Guide to GMP for Medicinal Products only require a company or organisation to nominate one person on a Manufacturer's Licence to carry out the duties of the Qualified Person provided that person is at the disposal of the company at all times and can carry out the required functions. However, an organisation may have either a complex structure, or operate at several locations, or both which would make it necessary for the company quality controller to delegate her/his duties to site staff. The Licensing Authority recognises that part of the quality control function involved with the assessment and authorisation of batches for despatch may require the organisation to nominate several Qualified Persons on its Manufacturer's Licence. Under these circumstances it may be desirable for the organisation not only to nominate an overall quality controller and site quality controller, but also to name both of them as Qualified Persons on the same licence to avoid confusion in line management responsibilities.

Where products are manufactured by an ML holder on behalf of a PL holder the arrangements for QP certification must be made clear in the contract. The contract receiver (the manufacturer) may accept that responsibility provided the QP has all the appropriate information and authority to fulfil these duties. Similarly, if the contract giver (when the PL holder is in a different organisation) chooses to employ her/his own QP, he/she must interpret her/his duties as laid down in the licence conditions to include arrangements for the QP to have access to all the appropriate information.

7.0 Delegation of Duties

7.1 The person responsible for Quality Control – who preferably should be a Qualified Person – should clearly define the areas of work and the method of deputising for absence for each Qualified Person.

7.2 Whilst each Qualified Person has a personal and professional responsibility for ensuring that the various checks and tests have been carried out, the detail of this work may be delegated to appropriately trained and experienced staff who would endorse their work. Confidence may be increased if the person to whom the work is delegated is also a member or a professional body bound by an ethical code of conduct. Ultimately the Qualified Person must be satisfied either directly or, more usually, by the proper operation of quality systems which include appropriate approvals, audits, self-inspections and spot checks that manufacturing and testing has complied with relevant requirements. Batch certification without such adequate steps is evidence of professional misconduct.

7.3 It must be recognised that the QP depends upon many of her/his working colleagues for the achievement of quality in the manufacture of medicinal products. It is therefore of paramount importance that he or she achieves a very good working relationship with other persons in positions of responsibility, especially the person responsible for production.

Other examples include those responsible for testing of materials and products and provision of engineering services who will also liaise closely with the QP in order to assist in the performance of his or her duties.

It is recommended that the company take the necessary steps to appraise other functional groups, and the responsible people who belong to them, of the importance attached to the role of the QP within the company and how they should give proper support.

7.4 The QP should be available at the manufacturing site for a sufficient proportion of the working time in order to be apprised of manufacturing conditions and for control of any delegation.

8.0 Education and Training

8.1 Qualified Persons have a personal and professional duty to keep their knowledge and experience up-to-date and in line with the current state of pharmaceutical quality management, product manufacturing and control technology, and general work practices. It is expected that appropriate records will be kept to reflect this important longer-term aspect of the QP's continued performance of professional duties.

8.2 In the event of a QP making a major change of job responsibilities, for example from a company making only sterile dose forms to one with a wider range of products including solid dose forms, then the QP and the top management of the company involved should recognise the possible need for additional education and training and take adequate steps to demonstrate that proper provision is made for this. (See also section 9.5(a) below)

9.0 Professional Code of Conduct

9.1 Qualified Persons are subject to the overall jurisdiction of the By-laws, Charters and Regulations, Codes of Conduct, Disciplinary Regulations and any general guidelines of the professional body, of which they are members, and should have access to them.

9.2 Qualified Persons have duties not only to their employer but also to the Licensing Authority and its Inspectorate. They must ensure through line management that appropriate senior company executives are fully aware of any manufacturing and/or testing difficulties which may cast doubt on the release of batches or post facto might require product recall.

If there is any aspect of the QA system which is not in accordance with the Directives and guidelines for Good Manufacturing Practice then the Qualified Person has a duty to bring this to the attention of Senior Management.

9.3 Qualified Persons should establish a good working relationship with MCA Inspectors and as far as possible provide information on request during site inspections.

9.4 The professional bodies verify (a) and (b) below when certifying the eligibility for nomination as a Qualified Person under the permanent provisions and the Licensing Authority accepts the relevant professional body's assessment of eligibility.

(a) The Qualified Person has demonstrated familiarity with all aspects of the knowledge of the Study Guide.

(b) The Qualified Person has satisfied the experience requirements as set out in the programme of practical experience.

9.5 The following assumptions are made, firstly by the professional bodies when certifying the eligibility of a Qualified Person and, secondly, by the Licensing Authority when accepting an eligible Qualified Person for nomination on a Manufacturer's Licence:

(a) In co-operation with their employers, Qualified Persons will take actions necessary to maintain and extend their technical and professional competence when they are engaged at a particular time.
(See also Section 8.0 above).

(b) In cases where undue pressures to depart from professional and technical standards cannot be counterbalanced by reference to this and other relevant Codes of Practice Qualified Persons, preferably having informed their employer first, should contact the appropriate professional body for confidential advice.

(c) Whilst management has a duty to provide Qualified Persons with appropriate resources and to ensure that systems and communication are working, Qualified Persons also have a duty to make representations to management, if necessary in writing, whenever standards appear to be falling short of Good Practice. This duty should be reflected by appropriate wording in the QP's job description.

10.0 Disciplinary Procedures

10.1 Directives 75/319/EEC and 81/851/EEC read inter alia-

"Member States shall ensure that the duties of Qualified Persons ... are fulfilled, either by means of appropriate administrative measures or by making such persons subject to a professional Code of Conduct".

"Member States may provide for the temporary suspension of such a person upon the commencement of administrative or disciplinary procedures against him for failure to fulfil his obligations".

10.2 SI 1977 No. 1053 reads inter alia–

"Where, after giving the licence holder and the person acting as a qualified person the opportunity of making representations to them (orally or in writing), the licensing authority are of the opinion that the person so acting does not satisfy the provisions of the said Articles 23 and 24 of the Second Council Directive as respects qualifications and experience, so that he is failing to carry out the functions specified ... and have notified the licence holder accordingly in writing, the licence holder shall not permit that person to act as a qualified person so long as the said notification has not been withdrawn by the licensing authority".

10.3 MAL 45 and MAL 69 read inter alia–

"The Qualified Person has a personal and professional responsibility for ensuring that the various tests and checks have been carried out. This does not necessarily mean that he/she must himself/herself have carried out those tests or have directly supervised them, but in certifying in the register or equivalent document he/she is in effect indicating that he/she has satisfied himself/herself that the appropriate tests have been carried out specifically for that batch and that batch complies with the relevant requirements. If it were found that a person had certified in such a register without taking adequate steps so to satisfy himself/herself, this failure might be a matter for consideration by the appropriate professional body to which he/she might belong as a matter of professional misconduct."

10.4 The professional bodies have established disciplinary machineries to deal with cases of possible misconduct. One of the powers is to remove the name of an individual from the appropriate register or registers and they will act together as appropriate in the case of a QP who is a member of two or three of the Societies. In such cases, professional bodies will inform the Licensing Authority, the body with the power to delete the Qualified Person's name from the Manufacturer's Licence.

11.0 Responsibility of Persons named on Manufacturer's Licences

Manufacturer's Licences contain the names of the persons responsible for Production, Quality Control, and the name(s) of the Qualified Person(s). The duties of these members of staff must be clear in their respective job descriptions and they must have the authority required under the relevant EC directives concerning medicinal products. In all cases the two sets of duties should be separately and clearly stated in job descriptions.

The responsibility for certifying that a product has been manufactured in accordance with its PL, with GMP and other requirements lies with the QP. Whilst the QP may not have line management responsibility for many activities he or she must be aware of any changes which may affect compliance with the PL or GMP before being asked to certify.

1993 (Revised)

Part Three

The GMP Directives 91/356/EEC and 91/341/EEC

EUROPEAN COMMISSION DIRECTIVES LAYING DOWN THE PRINCIPLES AND GUIDELINES OF GOOD MANUFACTURING PRACTICE

[**Note:** there are two Directives giving the principles and guidelines of good manufacturing practice (GMP), one for medicinal products for human use (Directive 91/356/EEC of 13 June 1992) and one for veterinary medicinal products (Directive 91/412/EEC of 23 July 1992). There are no differences of GMP between them, the main difference being in the cross-references to other Directives. The latest dates by which the Commission requires compliance are also different, being January 1992 and 23 July 1993 respectively.

For convenience of comparison, only one text is reproduced below but with the content of the veterinary Directive, where different from the human use Directive, italicised and in parenthesis eg. common and human-use text *(veterinary only text)*.]

Commission Directive of 13 July *(23 July)* 1991 laying down the principles and guidelines of good manufacturing practice for medicinal products for human use (91/356/EEC) (*veterinary medicinal products*) (*91/412/EEC*)

The Commission of the European Communities,

Having regard to the Treaty establishing the European Economic Community,

Having regard to Council Directive 75/319/EEC of 20 May 1975 on the approximation of provisions laid down by law, regulation or administrative action relating to proprietary medicinal products, as last amended by Directive 89/381/EEC, and in particular Article 19a thereof,

(Having regard to Council Directive 81/851/EEC of 28 September 1981 concerning the approximation of the laws of the Member States relating to veterinary medicinal products, as last amended by Directive 90/676/EEC, and in particular Article 27a,

Having regard to Council Directive 90/677/EEC of 13 December 1990 extending the scope of Directive 81/851/EEC on the approximation of the laws of the Member States relating to veterinary medicinal products and laying down additional provisions for immunological veterinary medicinal veterinary medicinal products,)

Whereas all medicinal products for human use *(veterinary medicinal products)* manufactured or imported into the Community, including medicinal products intended for export, should be manufactured in accordance with the principles and guidelines of good manufacturing practice;

Whereas, in accordance with national legislation, Member States may require compliance with these principles of good manufacturing practice during the manufacture of products intended for use in clinical trials;

Whereas the detailed guidelines mentioned in Article 19a of Directive 75/319/EEC (*27a of Directive 81/851/EEC*) have been published by the Commission after consultation with the pharmaceutical inspection services of the Member States in the form of a 'Guide to good manufacturing practice for medicinal products';

Whereas it is necessary that all manufacturers should operate an effective quality management of their manufacturing operations, and that this requires the implementation of a pharmaceutical quality assurance system;

Whereas officials representing the competent authorities should report on whether the manufacturer complies with good manufacturing practice and that these reports should be communicated upon reasoned request to the competent authorities of another Member State;

Whereas the principles and guidelines of good manufacturing practice should primarily concern personnel, premises and equipment, documentation, production, quality control, contracting out, complaints and product recall, and self inspection;

Whereas the principles and guidelines envisaged by this Directive are in accordance *(conformity)* with the opinion of the Committee for the Adaptation to Technical Progress of the Directives on the Removal of Technical Barriers to Trade in the Proprietary *(Veterinary)* Medicinal Products Sector set up by Article 2b of Council Directive 75/318/EEC *(81/852/EEC)* of 20 May 1975 *(28 September 1981)* on *(concerning)* the approximation of the laws of Member States relating to analytical, pharmaco-toxicological and clinical standards and protocols in respect of the testing of proprietary *(veterinary)* medicinal products, as last amended by Directive 89/341/EEC *(87/20/EEC),*

has adopted this directive

Chapter I

General Provisions

Article 1

This Directive lays down the principles and guidelines of good manufacturing practice for *(veterinary)* medicinal products whose manufacture requires the authorization referred to in Article 16 of Directive 75/319/EEC *(Article 24 of Directive 81/851/EEC).*

Article 2

For the purposes of this Directive, the definition of medicinal products set out in Article 1 (2) of Council Directive 65/65/EEC (5), *(and the definition of veterinary medicinal products set out in Article 1 (2) of Directive 81/851/EEC),* shall apply.

In addition,

– 'manufacturer' shall mean any holder of the authorization referred to in Article 16 of Directive 75/319/EEC *(Article 24 of Directive 81/851/EEC)*,

– 'qualified person' shall mean the person referred to in Article 21 of Directive 75/319/EEC *(Article 29 of Directive 81/851/EEC)*,

– 'pharmaceutical quality assurance' shall mean the sum total of the organized arrangements made with the object of ensuring that *(veterinary)* medicinal products are of the quality required for their intended use,

– 'good manufacturing practice' shall mean the part of quality `assurance which ensures that products are consistently produced and controlled to the quality standards appropriate to their intended use.

By means of the repeated inspections referred to in Article 26 of Directive 75/319/EEC *(Article 34 of Directive 81/851/EEC)*, the Member States shall ensure that manufacturers respect the principles and guidelines of good manufacturing practice laid down by this Directive.

For the interpretation of these principles and guidelines of good manufacturing practice, the manufacturers and the agents of the competent authorities shall refer to the detailed guidelines referred to in Article 19a of Directive 75/319/EEC *(Article 27a of Directive 81/851/EEC)*. These detailed guidelines are published by the Commission in the 'Guide to good manufacturing practice for medicinal products' and in its Annexes (Office for Official Publications of the European Communities, The rules governing medicinal products in the European Community, Volume IV).

Article 4

The manufacturer shall ensure that the manufacturing operations are carried out in accordance with good manufacturing practice and with the manufacturing authorization.

For *(veterinary)* medicinal products imported from third countries, the importer shall ensure that the *(veterinary)* medicinal products have been manufactured by manufacturers duly authorized and conforming to good manufacturing practice standards, at least equivalent to those laid down by the Community.

Article 5

The manufacturer shall ensure that all manufacturing operations subject to an authorization for marketing are carried out in accordance with the information given in the application for marketing authorization as accepted by the competent authorities.

The manufacturer shall regularly review their manufacturing methods in the light of scientific and technical progress. When a modification to the marketing authorization dossier is necessary, the application for modification must be submitted to the competent authorities.

Chapter II

Principles and Guidelines of Good Manufacturing Practice

Article 6

Quality management

The manufacturer shall establish and implement an effective pharmaceutical quality assurance system, involving the active participation of the management and personnel of the different services involved.

Article 7

Personnel

1. At each manufacturing site, the manufacturer shall have competent and appropriately qualified personnel at his disposal in sufficient number to achieve the pharmaceutical quality assurance objective(*s*).

2. The duties of managerial and supervisory staff, including the qualified person(s), responsible for implementing and operating good manufacturing practice shall be defined in job descriptions. Their hierarchical relationships shall be defined in an organization(*al*) chart. Organization*(al)* charts and job descriptions shall be approved in accordance with the manufacturer's internal procedures.

3. Staff referred to in paragraph 2 shall be given sufficient authority to discharge (*carry out*) their responsibilities correctly.

4. Personnel shall receive initial and continuing training including the theory and application of the concept of quality assurance and good manufacturing practice.

5. Hygiene programmes adapted to the activities to be carried out shall be established and observed. These programmes include procedures relating to health, hygiene and clothing of personnel.

Article 8

Premises and equipment

1. Premises and manufacturing equipment shall be located, designed, constructed, adapted and maintained to suit the intended operations.

2. Lay out, design and operation must aim to minimize the risk of errors and permit effective cleaning and maintenance in order to avoid contamination, cross contamination and, in general, any adverse effect on the quality of the product.

3. Premises and equipment intended to be used for manufacturing operations which are critical for the quality of the products shall be subjected to appropriate qualification.

Article 9

Documentation

1. The manufacturer shall have a system of documentation based upon specifications, manufacturing formulae and processing and packaging instructions, procedures and

records covering the various manufacturing operations that they perform. Documents shall be clear, free from errors and kept up to date. Pre-established procedures for general manufacturing operations and conditions shall be available, together with specific documents for the manufacture of each batch. This set of documents shall make it possible to trace the history of the manufacture of each batch. The batch documentation shall be retained for at least one year after the expiry date of the batches to which it relates or at least five years after the certification referred to in Article 22(2) of Directive 75/319/EEC *(Article 30(2) of Directive 81/851/EEC)* whichever is the longer.

2. When electronic, photographic or other data processing systems are used instead of written documents, the manufacturer shall have validated the systems by proving that the data will be appropriately stored during the anticipated period of storage. Data stored by these systems shall be made readily available in legible form. The electronically stored data shall be protected against loss or damage of data (eg by duplication or back-up and transfer onto another storage system).

Article 10

Production

The different production operations shall be carried out according to pre-established instructions and procedures and in accordance with good manufacturing practice. Adequate and sufficient resources shall be made available for the in-process controls.

Appropriate technical and/or organizational measures shall be taken to avoid cross contamination and mix-ups.

Any new manufacture or important modification of a manufacturing process shall be validated. Critical phases of manufacturing processes shall be regularly revalidated.

Article 11

Quality control

1. The manufacturer shall establish and maintain a quality control department. This department shall be placed under the authority of a person having the required qualifications and shall be independent of the other departments.

2. The quality control department shall have at its disposal one or more quality control laboratories appropriately staffed and equipped to carry out the necessary examination and testing of starting materials, packaging materials and intermediate and finished products testing. Resorting to outside laboratories may be authorized in accordance with Article 12 of this Directive after the authorization referred to in Article 5b of Directive 75/319/EEC *(Article 10(2) of Directive 81/851/EEC)* has been granted.

3. During the final control of finished products before their release for sale or distribution, in addition to analytical results, the quality control department shall take into account essential information such as the production conditions, the results of in-

process controls, the examination of the manufacturing documents and the conformity of the products to their specifications (including the final finished pack).

4. Samples of each batch of finished products shall be retained for at least one year after the expiry date. Unless in the Member States *(State)* of manufacture a longer period is required, samples of starting materials (other than solvents, gases and water) used shall be retained for at least two years after the release of the product. This period may be shortened if their stability, as mentioned in the relevant specification, is shorter. All these samples shall be maintained at the disposal of the competent authorities.

For certain *(veterinary)* medicinal products manufactured individually or in small quantities, or when their storage could raise special problems, other sampling and retaining conditions may be defined in agreement with the competent authority.

Article 12

Work contracted out

1. Any manufacturing operation or operation linked with the manufacture which is carried out under contract, shall be the subject of a written contract between the contract giver and the contract acceptor.

2. The contract shall clearly define the responsibilities of each party and in particular the observance of good manufacturing practice by the contract acceptor and the manner in which the qualified person responsible for releasing each batch shall undertake his full responsibilities.

3. The contract acceptor shall not subcontract any of the work entrusted to him by the contract giver without the written authorization of the contract giver.

4. The contract acceptor shall respect the principles and guidelines of good manufacturing practice and shall submit to inspections carried out by the competent authorities as provided for by Article 26 of Directive 75/319/EEC *(Article 34 of Directive 81/851/EEC)*.

Article 13

Complaints and product recall

The manufacturer shall implement a system for recording and reviewing complaints together with an effective system for recalling promptly and at any time the *(veterinary)* medicinal products in the distribution network. Any complaint concerning a defect shall be recorded and investigated by the manufacturer. The competent authority shall be informed by the manufacturer of any defect that could result in a recall or abnormal restriction on the supply. In so far as possible, the countries of destination shall also be indicated. Any recall shall be made in accordance with the requirements referred to in Article 33 of Directive 75/319/EEC *(Article 42 of Directive 81/851/EEC)*.

Article 14

Self-inspection
The manufacturer shall conduct repeated self-inspections as part of the quality assurance system in order to monitor the implementation and respect of good manufacturing practice and to propose any necessary corrective measures. Records of such self-inspections and any subsequent *(further)* corrective action shall be maintained.

Chapter III

Final Provisions

Article 15

Member States shall bring into force the laws, regulations and administrative provisions necessary to comply with this Directive not later than 1 January 1992 *(before 23 July 1993).* They shall forthwith inform the Commission thereof.

When Member States adopt these provisions, these shall contain a reference to this Directive or shall be accompanied by such reference at the time of their official publication. The procedure for such reference shall be adopted by Member States.

Article 16

This Directive is addressed to the Member States.

Done at Brussels, 13 June 1991 *(23 July 1991).*

Part Four

Guide to good manufacturing practice for medicinal products

INTRODUCTION

The Pharmaceutical Industry of the European Community maintains high standards of Quality Assurance in the development, manufacture and control of medicinal products. A system of Marketing Authorizations ensures that all medicinal products are assessed by a Competent Authority to ensure compliance with contemporary requirements of safety, quality and efficacy. A system of Manufacturing Authorizations ensures that all products authorized on the European market are manufactured only by authorized manufacturers, whose activities are regularly inspected by the Competent Authorities. Manufacturing Authorizations are required by all pharmaceutical manufacturers in the European Community whether the products are sold within or outside of the Community.

Two directives laying down principles and guidelines of good manufacturing practice (GMP) for medicinal products were adopted by the Commission in 1991, the first for medicinal products for human use (Directive 91/356/EEC), the second one for veterinary use (Directive 91/412/EEC). Detailed guidelines in accordance with those principles are published in the Guide to Good Manufacturing Practice which will be used in assessing applications for Manufacturing Authorizations and as a basis for inspection of manufacturers of medicinal products.

The principles of GMP and the detailed guidelines are applicable to all operations which require the authorization referred to in Article 16 of Directive 75/319/EEC and in Article 24 of Directive /851/EEC as modified. They are also relevant for all other large scale pharmaceutical manufacturing processes, such as that undertaken in hospitals, for the preparation of products for use in clinical trials, and for wholesaling, where applicable.

All Member States and the Industry itself are agreed that the GMP requirements applicable to the manufacture of veterinary medicinal products are the same as those applicable to the manufacture of medicinal products for human use. Certain detailed adjustments to the GMP guidelines are set out in two annexes specific to veterinary medicinal products and to immunological veterinary medicinal products.

The Guide is presented in chapters, each headed by a principle. Chapter 1 on Quality Management outlines the fundamental concept of Quality Assurance as applied to the manufacture of medicinal products. Thereafter each chapter has a principle outlining the Quality Assurance objectives of that chapter and a text which provides sufficient detail for manufacturers to be made aware of the essential matters to be considered when implementing the principle.

In addition to the general matters of Good Manufacturing Practice outlined in the 9 chapters of this guide, a series of annexes providing detail about specific areas of activity is included. For some manufacturing processes, different annexes will apply simultaneously (e.g. annex on sterile preparations and on radiopharmaceuticals and/or on biological medicinal products).

CONTENTS

Basic Requirements

CHAPTER 1: QUALITY MANAGEMENT 47
Principle 47
Quality Assurance 47
Good Manufacturing Practice for Medicinal Products 48
Quality Control 49

CHAPTER 2: PERSONNEL 51
Principle 51
General 51
Key Personnel 51
Training 53
Personnel Hygiene 53

CHAPTER 3: PREMISES AND EQUIPMENT 55
Principle 55
Premises 55
General 55
Production Area 55
Storage Area 57
Quality Control Area 57
Ancillary Area 58
Equipment 58

CHAPTER 4: DOCUMENTATION 61
Principle 61
General 61
Documents Required 62
Specifications 62
Starting and Packaging Materials 62
Intermediate and Bulk Products 63
Finished Products 63
Manufacturing Formula and Processing Instructions 63
Packaging Instructions 64
Batch Processing Records 64
Batch Packaging Records 65
Procedures and Records 66
Receipt 66

Sampling 66
Testing 66
Other 41 66

CHAPTER 5: PRODUCTION 69
Principle 69
General 69
Prevention of Cross-contamination in Production 70
Validation 71
Starting Materials 71
Processing Operations: Intermediate and Bulk Products 72
Packaging Materials 72
Packaging Operations 73
Finished Products 74
Rejected, Recovered and Returned Materials 74

CHAPTER 6: QUALITY CONTROL 77
Principle 77
General 77
Good Quality Control Laboratory Practice 77
Documentation 78
Sampling 78
Testing 79

CHAPTER 7: CONTRACT MANUFACTURE AND ANALYSIS 81
Principle 81
General 81
The Contract Giver 81
The Contract Acceptor 82
The Contract 82

CHAPTER 8: COMPLAINTS AND PRODUCT RECALL 85
Principle 85
Complaints 85
Recalls 85

CHAPTER 9: SELF INSPECTION 87
Principle 87

ANNEXES 89
1. Manufacture of sterile medicinal products 91
2. Manufacture of biological medicinal products for human use 103
3. Manufacture of radiopharmaceuticals 111
4. Manufacture of veterinary medicinal products other than immunologicals 113
5. Manufacture of immunological veterinary medicinal products 115
6. Manufacture of medicinal gases 127

7. Manufacture of herbal medicinal products 131
8. Sampling of starting and packaging materials 135
9. Manufacture of liquids, creams and ointments 137
10. Manufacture of pressurized metered dose aerosol preparations for inhalation 139
11. Computerized systems 141
12. Use of ionizing radiation in the manufacture of medicinal products 145
13. Good manufacturing practice for investigational medicinal products 153
14. Manufacture of products derived from human blood or human plasma 163

GLOSSARY 169

SUBJECT INDEX 177

Basic Requirements

1 QUALITY MANAGEMENT

Principle

The holder of a Manufacturing Authorization must manufacture medicinal products so as to ensure that they are fit for their intended use, comply with the requirements of the Marketing Authorization and do not place patients at risk due to inadequate safety, quality or efficacy. The attainment of this quality objective is the responsibility of senior management and requires the participation and commitment by staff in many different departments and at all levels within the company, by the company's suppliers and by the distributors. To achieve the quality objective reliably there must be a comprehensively designed and correctly implemented system of Quality Assurance incorporating Good Manufacturing Practice and thus Quality Control. It should be fully documented and its effectiveness monitored. All parts of the Quality Assurance system should be adequately resourced with competent personnel, and suitable and sufficient premises, equipment and facilities. There are additional legal responsibilities for the holder of the Manufacturing Authorisation and for the Qualified Person(s).

1.1. The basic concepts of Quality Assurance, Good Manufacturing Practice and Quality Control are inter-related. They are described here in order to emphasise their relationships and their fundamental importance to the production and control of medicinal products.

Quality Assurance

1.2. Quality Assurance is a wide ranging concept which covers all matters which individually or collectively influence the quality of a product. It is the sum total of the organised arrangements made with the object of ensuring that medicinal products are of the quality required for their intended use. Quality Assurance therefore incorporates Good Manufacturing Practice plus other factors outside the scope of this Guide.

The system of Quality Assurance appropriate for the manufacture of medicinal products should ensure that:

i. medicinal products are designed and developed in a way that takes account of the requirements of Good Manufacturing Practice and Good Laboratory Practice;

ii. production and control operations are clearly specified and Good Manufacturing Practice adopted;

iii. managerial responsibilities are clearly specified;

iv. arrangements are made for the manufacture, supply and use of the correct starting and packaging materials;

v. all necessary controls on intermediate products, and any other in-process controls and validations are carried out;

vi. the finished product is correctly processed and checked, according to the defined procedures;

vii. medicinal products are not sold or supplied before a Qualified Person has certified that each production batch has been produced and controlled in accordance with the requirements of the Marketing Authorisation and any other regulations relevant to the production, control and release of medicinal products;

viii. satisfactory arrangements exist to ensure, as far as possible, that the medicinal products are stored, distributed and subsequently handled so that quality is maintained throughout their shelf life;

ix. there is a procedure for Self-Inspection and/or quality audit which regularly appraises the effectiveness and applicability of the Quality Assurance system.

Good Manufacturing Practice for Medicinal Products (GMP)

1.3. Good Manufacturing Practice is that part of Quality Assurance which ensures that products are consistently produced and controlled to the quality standards appropriate to their intended use and as required by the Marketing Authorisation or product specification.

Good Manufacturing Practice is concerned with both production and quality control. The basic requirements of GMP are that:

i. all manufacturing processes are clearly defined, systematically reviewed in the light of experience and shown to be capable of consistently manufacturing medicinal products of the required quality and complying with their specifications;

ii. critical steps of manufacturing processes and significant changes to the process are validated;

iii. all necessary facilities for GMP are provided including:

a. appropriately qualified and trained personnel;

b. adequate premises and space;

c. suitable equipment and services;

d. correct materials, containers and labels;

e. approved procedures and instructions;

f. suitable storage and transport;

iv. instructions and procedures are written in an instructional form in clear and unambiguous language, specifically applicable to the facilities provided;
v. operators are trained to carry out procedures correctly;
vi. records are made, manually and/or by recording instruments, during manufacture which demonstrate that all the steps required by the defined procedures and instructions were in fact taken and that the quantity and quality of the product was as expected. Any significant deviations are fully recorded and investigated;
vii. records of manufacture including distribution which enable the complete history of a batch to be traced, are retained in a comprehensible and accessible form;
viii. the distribution (wholesaling) of the products minimises any risk to their quality;
ix. a system is available to recall any batch of product, from sale or supply;
x. complaints about marketed products are examined, the causes of quality defects investigated and appropriate measures taken in respect of the defective products and to prevent reoccurrence.

Quality Control

1.4. Quality Control is that part of Good Manufacturing Practice which is concerned with sampling, specifications and testing, and with the organisation, documentation and release procedures which ensure that the necessary and relevant tests are actually carried out and that materials are not released for use, nor products released for sale or supply, until their quality has been judged to be satisfactory.

The basic requirements of Quality Control are that:

i. adequate facilities, trained personnel and approved procedures are available for sampling, inspecting and testing starting materials, packaging materials, intermediate, bulk, and finished products, and where appropriate for monitoring environmental conditions for GMP purposes;
ii. samples of starting materials, packaging materials, intermediate products, bulk products and finished products are taken by personnel and by methods approved by Quality Control;
iii. test methods are validated;
iv. records are made, manually and/or by recording instruments, which demonstrate that all the required sampling, inspecting and testing procedures were actually carried out. Any deviations are fully recorded and investigated;
v. the finished products contain active ingredients complying with the qualitative and quantitative composition of the Marketing Authorisation, are of the purity required, and are enclosed within their proper containers and correctly labelled;

vi. records are made of the results of inspection and that testing of materials, intermediate, bulk, and finished products is formally assessed against specification. Product assessment includes a review and evaluation of relevant production documentation and an assessment of deviations from specified procedures;

vii. no batch of product is released for sale or supply prior to certification by a Qualified Person that it is in accordance with the requirements of the Marketing Authorization;

viii. sufficient reference samples of starting materials and products are retained to permit future examination of the product if necessary and that the product is retained in its final pack unless exceptionally large packs are produced.

2 PERSONNEL

Principle

The establishment and maintenance of a satisfactory system of quality assurance and the correct manufacture of medicinal products relies upon people. For this reason there must be sufficient qualified personnel to carry out all the tasks which are the responsibility of the manufacturer. Individual responsibilities should be clearly understood by the individuals and recorded. All personnel should be aware of the principles of Good Manufacturing Practice that affect them and receive initial and continuing training, including hygiene instructions, relevant to their needs.

General

2.1. The manufacturer should have an adequate number of personnel with the necessary qualifications and practical experience. The responsibilities placed on any one individual should not be so extensive as to present any risk to quality.

2.2. The manufacturer must have an organization chart. People in responsible positions should have specific duties recorded in written job descriptions and adequate authority to carry out their responsibilities. Their duties may be delegated to designated deputies of a satisfactory qualification level. There should be no gaps or unexplained overlaps in the responsibilities of those personnel concerned with the application of Good Manufacturing Practice.

Key Personnel

2.3. Key Personnel include the head of Production, the head of Quality Control, and if at least one of these persons is not responsible for the duties described in Article 22 of Directive 75/319/EEC, the Qualified Person(s) designated for the purpose. Normally key posts should be occupied by full-time personnel. The heads of Production and Quality Control must be independent from each other. In large organisations, it may be necessary to delegate some of the functions listed in 2.5., 2.6. and 2.7.

2.4. The duties of the Qualified Person(s) are fully described in Article 22 of Directive 75/319/EEC, and can be summarised as follows:

(a) for medicinal products manufactured within the European Community, a Qualified Person must ensure that each batch has been produced and tested/checked in accordance with the directives and the marketing authorisation(*);

(*) According to Directive 75/319/EEC and the Ruling (Case 247/81) of the Court of Justice of the European Communities, medicinal products which have been properly controlled in the EEC by a Qualified Person do not have to be recontrolled or rechecked in any other Member State of the Community.

(b) for medicinal products manufactured outside the European Community, a Qualified Person must ensure that each imported batch has undergone, in the importing country, the testing specified in paragraph 1 (b) of Article 22;

(c) a Qualified Person must certify in a register or equivalent document, as operations are carried out and before any release, that each production batch satisfies the provisions of Article 22.

The persons responsible for these duties must meet the qualification requirements laid down in Article 23 of the same Directive, they shall be permanently and continuously at the disposal of the holder of the Manufacturing Authorization to carry out their responsibilities. Their responsibilities may be delegated, but only to other Qualified Person(s).

2.5. The head of the Production Department generally has the following responsibilities:

i. to ensure that products are produced and stored according to the appropriate documentation in order to obtain the required quality;
ii. to approve the instructions relating to production operations and to ensure their strict implementation;
iii. to ensure that the production records are evaluated and signed by an authorised person before they are sent to the Quality Control Department;
iv. to check the maintenance of his department, premises and equipment;
v. to ensure that the appropriate validations are done;
vi. to ensure that the required initial and continuing training of his department personnel is carried out and adapted according to need.

2.6. The head of the Quality Control Department generally has the following responsibilities:

i. to approve or reject, as he sees fit, starting materials, packaging materials, and intermediate, bulk and finished products;
ii. to evaluate batch records;
iii. to ensure that all necessary testing is carried out;
iv. to approve specifications, sampling instructions, test methods and other Quality Control procedures;
v. to approve and monitor any contract analysts;
vi. to check the maintenance of his department, premises and equipment;
vii. to ensure that the appropriate validations are done;
viii. to ensure that the required initial and continuing training of his department personnel is carried out and adapted according to need.

Other duties of the Quality Control Department are summarized in Chapter 6.

2.7. The heads of Production and Quality Control generally have some shared, or jointly exercised, responsibilities relating to quality. These may include, subject to any national regulations:

- the authorisation of written procedures and other documents, including amendments;

- the monitoring and control of the manufacturing environment;
- plant hygiene;
- process validation;
- training;
- the approval and monitoring of suppliers of materials;
- the approval and monitoring of contract manufacturers;
- the designation and monitoring of storage conditions for materials and products;
- the retention of records;
- the monitoring of compliance with the requirements of Good Manufacturing Practice;
- the inspection, investigation, and taking of samples, in order to monitor factors which may affect product quality.

Training

2.8. The manufacturer should provide training for all the personnel whose duties take them into production areas or into control laboratories (including the technical, maintenance and cleaning personnel), and for other personnel whose activities could affect the quality of the product.

2.9. Besides the basic training on the theory and practice of Good Manufacturing Practice, newly recruited personnel should receive training appropriate to the duties assigned to them. Continuing training should also be given, and its practical effectiveness should be periodically assessed. Training programs should be available, approved by either the head of Production or the head of Quality Control, as appropriate. Training records should be kept.

2.10. Personnel working in areas where contamination is a hazard, e.g. clean areas or areas where highly active, toxic, infectious or sensitizing materials are handled, should be given specific training.

2.11. Visitors or untrained personnel should, preferably, not be taken into the production and quality control areas. If this is unavoidable, they should be given information in advance, particularly about personal hygiene and the prescribed protective clothing. They should be closely supervised.

2.12. The concept of Quality Assurance and all the measures capable of improving its understanding and implementation should be fully discussed during the training sessions.

Personnel Hygiene

2.13. Detailed hygiene programmes should be established and adapted to the different needs within the factory. They should include procedures relating to the health, hygiene practices and clothing of personnel. These procedures should be understood and followed in a very strict way by every person whose duties take him into the production and control areas. Hygiene programmes should be promoted by management and widely discussed during training sessions.

2.14. All personnel should receive medical examination upon recruitment. It must be the manufacturer's responsibility that there are instructions ensuring that health conditions that can be of relevance to the quality of products come to the manufacturer's knowledge. After the first medical examination, examinations should be carried out when necessary for the work and personal health.

2.15. Steps should be taken to ensure as far as is practicable that no person affected by an infectious disease or having open lesions on the exposed surface of the body is engaged in the manufacture of medicinal products.

2.16. Every person entering the manufacturing areas should wear protective garments appropriate to the operations to be carried out.

2.17. Eating, drinking, chewing or smoking, or the storage of food, drink, smoking materials or personal medication in the production and storage areas should be prohibited. In general, any unhygienic practice within the manufacturing areas or in any other area where the product might be adversely affected, should be forbidden.

2.18. Direct contact should be avoided between the operator's hands and the exposed product as well as with any part of the equipment that comes into contact with the products.

2.19. Personnel should be instructed to use the hand-washing facilities.

2.20. Any specific requirements for the manufacture of special groups of products, for example sterile preparations, are covered in the annexes.

3 PREMISES AND EQUIPMENT

Principle

Premises and equipment must be located, designed, constructed, adapted and maintained to suit the operations to be carried out. Their layout and design must aim to minimize the risk of errors and permit effective cleaning and maintenance in order to avoid cross-contamination, build up of dust or dirt and, in general, any adverse effect on the quality of products.

PREMISES

General

3.1. Premises should be situated in an environment which, when considered together with measures to protect the manufacture, presents minimal risk of causing contamination of materials or products.

3.2. Premises should be carefully maintained, ensuring that repair and maintenance operations do not present any hazard to the quality of products. They should be cleaned and, where applicable, disinfected according to detailed written procedures.

3.3. Lighting, temperature, humidity and ventilation should be appropriate and such that they do not adversely affect, directly or indirectly, either the medicinal products during their manufacture and storage, or the accurate functioning of equipment.

3.4. Premises should be designed and equipped so as to afford maximum protection against the entry of insects or other animals.

3.5. Steps should be taken in order to prevent the entry of unauthorized people. Production, storage and quality control areas should not be used as a right of way by personnel who do not work in them.

Production Area

3.6. In order to minimize the risk of a serious medical hazard due to cross-contamination, dedicated and self contained facilities must be available for the production of particular medicinal products, such as highly sensitizing materials (e.g. penicillins) or biological preparations (e.g. from live micro-organisms). The production of certain additional products, such as certain antibiotics, certain hormones, certain cytotoxics, certain highly active drugs and non-medicinal products should not be conducted in the same facilities. For those products, in exceptional cases, the principle of campaign working in the same facilities can be accepted provided that specific precautions are taken and the necessary validations are made. The manufacture of technical poisons, such as pesticides and herbicides, should not be allowed in premises used for the manufacture of medicinal products.

3.7. Premises should preferably be laid out in such a way as to allow the production to take place in areas connected in a logical order corresponding to the sequence of the operations and to the requisite cleanliness levels.

3.8. The adequacy of the working and in-process storage space should permit the orderly and logical positioning of equipment and materials so as to minimize the risk of confusion between different medicinal products or their components, to avoid cross-contamination and to minimize the risk of omission or wrong application of any of the manufacturing or control steps.

3.9. Where starting and primary packaging materials, intermediate or bulk products are exposed to the environment, interior surfaces (walls, floors and ceilings) should be smooth, free from cracks and open joints, and should not shed particulate matter and should permit easy and effective cleaning and, if necessary, disinfection.

3.10. Pipework, light fittings, ventilation points and other services should be designed and sited to avoid the creation of recesses which are difficult to clean. As far as possible, for maintenance purposes, they should be accessible from outside the manufacturing areas.

3.11. Drains should be of adequate size, and have trapped gullies. Open channels should be avoided where possible, but if necessary, they should be shallow to facilitate cleaning and disinfection.

3.12. Production areas should be effectively ventilated, with air control facilities (including temperature and, where necessary, humidity and filtration) appropriate both to the products handled, to the operations undertaken within them and to the external environment.

3.13. Weighing of starting materials usually should be carried out in a separate weighing room designed for that use.

3.14. In cases where dust is generated (e.g. during sampling, weighing, mixing and processing operations, packaging of dry products), specific provisions should be taken to avoid cross-contamination and facilitate cleaning.

3.15. Premises for the packaging of medicinal products should be specifically designed and laid out so as to avoid mix-ups or cross-contamination.

3.16. Production areas should be well lit, particularly where visual on-line controls are carried out.

3.17. In-process controls may be carried out within the production area provided they do not carry any risk for the production.

Storage Areas

3.18. Storage areas should be of sufficient capacity to allow orderly storage of the various categories of materials and products: starting and packaging materials, intermediate, bulk and finished products, products in quarantine, released, rejected, returned or recalled.

3.19. Storage areas should be designed or adapted to ensure good storage conditions. In particular, they should be clean and dry and maintained within acceptable temperature limits. Where special storage conditions are required (e.g. temperature, humidity) these should be provided, checked and monitored.

3.20. Receiving and dispatch bays should protect materials and products from the weather. Reception areas should be designed and equipped to allow containers of incoming materials to be cleaned where necessary before storage.

3.21. Where quarantine status is ensured by storage in separate areas, these areas must be clearly marked and their access restricted to authorized personnel. Any system replacing the physical quarantine should give equivalent security.

3.22. There should normally be a separate sampling area for starting materials. If sampling is performed in the storage area, it should be conducted in such a way as to prevent contamination or cross-contamination.

3.23. Segregated areas should be provided for the storage of rejected, recalled or returned materials or products.

3.24. Highly active materials or products should be stored in safe and secure areas.

3.25. Printed packaging materials are considered critical to the conformity of the medicinal product and special attention should be paid to the safe and secure storage of these materials.

Quality Control Areas

3.26. Normally, Quality Control laboratories should be separated from production areas. This is particularly important for laboratories for the control of biologicals, microbiologicals and radioisotopes, which should also be separated from each other.

3.27. Control laboratories should be designed to suit the operations to be carried out in them. Sufficient space should be given to avoid mix-ups and cross-contamination. There should be adequate suitable storage space for samples and records.

3.28. Separate rooms may be necessary to protect sensitive instruments from vibration, electrical interference, humidity, etc.

3.29. Special requirements are needed in laboratories handling particular substances, such as biological or radioactive samples.

Ancillary Areas

3.30. Rest and refreshment rooms should be separate from other areas.

3.31. Facilities for changing clothes, and for washing and toilet purposes should be easily accessible and appropriate for the number of users. Toilets should not directly communicate with production or storage areas.

3.32. Maintenance workshops should as far as possible be separate from production areas. Whenever parts and tools are stored in the production area, they should be kept in rooms or lockers reserved for that use.

3.33. Animal houses should be well isolated from other areas, with separate entrance (animal access) and air handling facilities.

Equipment

3.34. Manufacturing equipment should be designed, located and maintained to suit its intended purpose.

3.35. Repair and maintenance operations should not present any hazard to the quality of the products.

3.36. Manufacturing equipment should be designed so that it can be easily and thoroughly cleaned. It should be cleaned according to detailed and written procedures and stored only in a clean and dry condition.

3.37. Washing and cleaning equipment should be chosen and used in order not to be a source of contamination.

3.38. Equipment should be installed in such a way as to prevent any risk of error or of contamination.

3.39. Production equipment should not present any hazard to the products. The parts of the production equipment that come into contact with the product must not be reactive, additive or absorptive to such an extent that it will affect the quality of the product and thus present any hazard.

3.40. Balances and measuring equipment of an appropriate range and precision should be available for production and control operations.

3.41. Measuring, weighing, recording and control equipment should be calibrated and checked at defined intervals by appropriate methods. Adequate records of such tests should be maintained.

3.42. Fixed pipework should be clearly labelled to indicate the contents and, where applicable, the direction of flow.

3.43. Distilled, deionized and, where appropriate, other water pipes should be sanitized according to written procedures that detail the action limits for microbiological contamination and the measures to be taken.

3.44. Defective equipment should, if possible, be removed from production and quality control areas, or at least be clearly labelled as defective.

4 DOCUMENTATION

Principle

Good documentation constitutes an essential part of the quality assurance system. Clearly written documentation prevents errors from spoken communication and permits tracing of batch history. Specifications, Manufacturing Formulae and Instructions, procedures, and records must be free from errors and available in writing. The legibility of documents is of paramount importance.

General

4.1. *Specifications* describe in detail the requirements with which the products or materials used or obtained during manufacture have to conform. They serve as a basis for quality evaluation.

Manufacturing Formulae, Processing and Packaging Instructions state all the starting materials used and lay down all processing and packaging operations.

Procedures give directions for performing certain operations eg cleaning, clothing, environmental control, sampling, testing, equipment operation.

Records provide a history of each batch of product, including its distribution, and also of all other relevant circumstances pertinent to the quality of the final product.

4.2. Documents should be designed, prepared, reviewed and distributed with care. They should comply with the relevant parts of the manufacturing and marketing authorization dossiers.

4.3. Documents should be approved, signed and dated by appropriate and authorized persons.

4.4. Documents should have unambiguous contents; title, nature and purpose should be clearly stated. They should be laid out in an orderly fashion and be easy to check. Reproduced documents should be clear and legible. The reproduction of working documents from master documents must not allow any error to be introduced through the reproduction process.

4.5. Documents should be regularly reviewed and kept up-to-date. When a document has been revised, systems should be operated to prevent inadvertent use of superseded documents.

4.6. Documents should not be handwritten; although, where documents require the entry of data, these entries may be made in clear, legible, indelible handwriting. Sufficient space should be provided for such entries.

4.7. Any alteration made to the entry on a document should be signed and dated; the alteration should permit the reading of the original information. Where appropriate, the reason for the alteration should be recorded.

4.8. The records should be made or completed at the time each action is taken and in such a way that all significant activities concerning the manufacture of medicinal products are traceable. They should be retained for at least one year after the expiry date of the finished product.

4.9. Data may be recorded by electronic data processing systems, photographic or other reliable means, but detailed procedures relating to the system in use should be available and the accuracy of the records should be checked. If documentation is handled by electronic data processing methods, only authorized persons should be able to enter or modify data in the computer and there should be a record of changes and deletions; access should be restricted by passwords or other means and the result of entry of critical data should be independently checked. Batch records electronically stored should be protected by back-up transfer on magnetic tape, microfilm, paper or other means. It is particularly important that the data are readily available throughout the period of retention.

Documents required

4.10. Specifications

There should be appropriately authorized and dated specifications for starting and packaging materials, and finished products; where appropriate, they should be also available for intermediate or bulk products.

Specifications for starting and packaging materials

4.11. Specifications for starting and primary or printed packaging materials should include, if applicable:

(a) a description of the materials, including:
- the designated name and the internal code reference;
- the reference, if any, to a pharmacopoeial monograph;
- the approved suppliers and, if possible, the original producer of the products;
- a specimen of printed materials;

(b) directions for sampling and testing or reference to procedures;

(c) qualitative and quantitative requirements with acceptance limits;

(d) storage conditions and precautions;

(e) the maximum period of storage before re-examination.

Specifications for intermediate and bulk products

4.12. Specifications for intermediate and bulk products should be available if these are purchased or dispatched, or if data obtained from intermediate products are used for the evaluation of the finished product. The specifications should be similar to specifications for starting materials or for finished products, as appropriate.

Specifications for finished products

4.13. Specifications for finished products should include:
- (a) the designated name of the product and the code reference where applicable;
- (b) the formula or a reference to;
- (c) a description of the pharmaceutical form and package details;
- (d) directions for sampling and testing or a reference to procedures;
- (e) the qualitative and quantitative requirements, with the acceptance limits;
- (f) the storage conditions and any special handling precautions, where applicable;
- (g) the shelf-life.

Manufacturing Formula and Processing Instructions

Formally authorized Manufacturing Formula and Processing Instructions should exist for each product and batch size to be manufactured. They are often combined in one document.

4.14. The Manufacturing Formula should include:
- (a) the name of the product, with a product reference code relating to its specification;
- (b) a description of the pharmaceutical form, strength of the product and batch size;
- (c) a list of all starting materials to be used, with the amount of each, described using the designated name and a reference which is unique to that material; mention should be made of any substance that may disappear in the course of processing;
- (d) a statement of the expected final yield with the acceptable limits, and of relevant intermediate yields, where applicable.

4.15. The Processing Instructions should include:
- (a) a statement of the processing location and the principal equipment to be used;
- (b) the methods, or reference to the methods, to be used for preparing the critical equipment (e.g. cleaning, assembling, calibrating, sterilising);
- (c) detailed stepwise processing instructions (e.g. checks on materials, pretreatments, sequence for adding materials, mixing times, temperatures);
- (d) the instructions for any in-process controls with their limits;
- (e) where necessary, the requirements for bulk storage of the products; including the container, labelling and special storage conditions where applicable;

(f) any special precautions to be observed.

Packaging Instructions

4.16. There should be formally authorized Packaging Instructions for each product, pack size and type. These should normally include, or have a reference to, the following:

(a) name of the product;

(b) description of its pharmaceutical form, and strength where applicable;

(c) the pack size expressed in terms of the number, weight or volume of the product in the final container;

(d) a complete list of all the packaging materials required for a standard batch size, including quantities, sizes and types, with the code or reference number relating to the specifications of each packaging material;

(e) where appropriate, an example or reproduction of the relevant printed packaging materials, and specimens indicating where to apply batch number references, and shelf life of the product;

(f) special precautions to be observed, including a careful examination of the area and equipment in order to ascertain the line clearance before operations begin;

(g) a description of the packaging operation, including any significant subsidiary operations, and equipment to be used;

(h) details of in-process controls with instructions for sampling and acceptance limits.

Batch Processing Records

4.17. A Batch Processing Record should be kept for each batch processed. It should be based on the relevant parts of the currently approved Manufacturing Formula and Processing Instructions. The method of preparation of such records should be designed to avoid transcription errors. The record should carry the number of the batch being manufactured.

Before any processing begins, there should be recorded checks that the equipment and work station are clear of previous products, documents or materials not required for the planned process, and that equipment is clean and suitable for use.

During processing, the following information should be recorded at the time each action is taken and, after completion, the record should be dated and signed in agreement by the person responsible for the processing operations:

(a) the name of the product;

(b) dates and times of commencement, of significant intermediate stages and of completion of production;

(c) name of the person responsible for each stage of production;

(d) initials of the operator of different significant steps of production and, where appropriate, of the person who checked each of these operations (e. g. weighing);
(e) the batch number and/or analytical control number as well as the quantities of each starting material actually weighed (including the batch number and amount of any recovered or reprocessed material added);
(f) any relevant processing operation or event and major equipment used;
(g) a record of the in-process controls and the initials of the person(s) carrying them out, and the results obtained;
(h) the product yield obtained at different and pertinent stages of manufacture;
(i) notes on special problems including details, with signed authorization for any deviation from the Manufacturing Formula and Processing Instructions.

Batch Packaging Records

4.18 A Batch Packaging Record should be kept for each batch or part batch processed. It should be based on the relevant parts of the Packaging Instructions and the method of preparation of such records should be designed to avoid transcription errors. The record should carry the batch number and the quantity of bulk product to be packed, as well as the batch number and the planned quantity of finished product that will be obtained.

Before any packaging operation begins, there should be recorded checks that the equipment and work station are clear of previous products, documents or materials not required for the planned packaging operations, and that equipment is clean and suitable for use.

The following information should be entered at the time each action is taken and, after completion, the record should be dated and signed in agreement by the person(s) responsible for the packaging operations:
(a) the name of the product;
(b) the date(s) and times of the packaging operations;
(c) the name of the responsible person carrying out the packaging operation;
(d) the initials of the operators of the different significant steps;
(e) records of checks for identity and conformity with the packaging instructions including the results of in-process controls;
(f) details of the packaging operations carried out, including references to equipment and the packaging lines used;
(g) whenever possible, samples of printed packaging materials used, including specimens of the batch coding, expiry dating and any additional overprinting;
(h) notes on any special problems or unusual events including details, with signed authorization for any deviation from the Manufacturing Formula and Processing Instructions;
(i) the quantities and reference number or identification of all printed packaging materials and bulk product issued, used, destroyed or returned to stock and

the quantities of obtained product, in order to provide for an adequate reconciliation.

Procedures and records

Receipt

4.19. There should be written procedures and records for the receipt of each delivery of each starting and primary and printed packaging material.

4.20. The records of the receipts should include:
- (a) the name of the material on the delivery note and the containers;
- (b) the "in-house" name and/or code of material (if different from a);
- (c) date of receipt;
- (d) supplier's name and, if possible, manufacturer's name;
- (e) manufacturer's batch or reference number;
- (f) total quantity, and number of containers received;
- (g) the batch number assigned after receipt;
- (h) any relevant comment (e.g. state of the containers).

4.21. There should be written procedures for the internal labelling, quarantine and storage of starting materials, packaging materials and other materials, as appropriate.

Sampling

4.22. There should be written procedures for sampling, which include the person(s) authorized to take samples, the methods and equipment to be used, the amounts to be taken and any precautions to be observed to avoid contamination of the material or any deterioration in its quality (see Chapter 6, item 13).

Testing

4.23. There should be written procedures for testing materials and products at different stages of manufacture, describing the methods and equipment to be used. The tests performed should be recorded (see Chapter 6, item 17).

Other

4.24. Written release and rejection procedures should be available for materials and products, and in particular for the release for sale of the finished product by the Qualified Person(s) in accordance with the requirements of Article 22 of Directive 75/319/EEC.

4.25. Records should be maintained of the distribution of each batch of a product in order to facilitate the recall of the batch if necessary (see Chapter 8).

4.26. There should be written procedures and the associated records of actions taken or conclusions reached, where appropriate, for:

- validation;
- equipment assembly and calibration;
- maintenance, cleaning and sanitization;
- personnel matters including training, clothing, hygiene;
- environmental monitoring;
- pest control;
- complaints;
- recalls;
- returns.

4.27. Clear operating procedures should be available for major items of manufacturing and test equipment.

4.28. Log books should be kept for major or critical equipment recording, as appropriate, any validations, calibrations, maintenance, cleaning or repair operations, including the dates and identity of people who carried these operations out.

4.29. Log books should also record in chronological order the use of major or critical equipment and the areas where the products have been processed.

5 PRODUCTION

Principle

Production operations must follow clearly defined procedures; they must comply with the principles of Good Manufacturing Practice in order to obtain products of the requisite quality and be in accordance with the relevant manufacturing and marketing authorizations.

General

5.1. Production should be performed and supervised by competent people.

5.2. All handling of materials and products, such as receipt and quarantine, sampling, storage, labelling, dispensing, processing, packaging and distribution should be done in accordance with written procedures or instructions and, where necessary, recorded.

5.3. All incoming materials should be checked to ensure that the consignment corresponds to the order. Containers should be cleaned where necessary and labelled with the prescribed data.

5.4. Damage to containers and any other problem which might adversely affect the quality of a material should be investigated, recorded and reported to the Quality Control Department.

5.5. Incoming materials and finished products should be physically or administratively quarantined immediately after receipt or processing, until they have been released for use or distribution.

5.6. Intermediate and bulk products purchased as such should be handled on receipt as though they were starting materials.

5.7. All materials and products should be stored under the appropriate conditions established by the manufacturer and in an orderly fashion to permit batch segregation and stock rotation.

5.8. Checks on yields, and reconciliation of quantities, should be carried out as necessary to ensure that there are no discrepancies outside acceptable limits.

5.9. Operations on different products should not be carried out simultaneously or consecutively in the same room unless there is no risk of mix-up or cross-contamination.

5.10. At every stage of processing, products and materials should be protected from microbial and other contamination.

5.11. When working with dry materials and products, special precautions should be taken to prevent the generation and dissemination of dust. This applies particularly to the handling of highly active or sensitizing materials.

5.12. At all times during processing, all materials, bulk containers, major items of equipment and where appropriate rooms used should be labelled or otherwise identified with an indication of the product or material being processed, its strength (where applicable) and batch number. Where applicable, this indication should also mention the stage of production.

5.13. Labels applied to containers, equipment or premises should be clear, unambiguous and in the company's agreed format. It is often helpful in addition to the wording on the labels to use colours to indicate status (for example, quarantined, accepted, rejected, clean, ...).

5.14. Checks should be carried out to ensure that pipelines and other pieces of equipment used for the transportation of products from one area to another are connected in a correct manner.

5.15. Any deviation from instructions or procedures should be avoided as far as possible. If a deviation occurs, it should be approved in writing by a competent person, with the involvement of the Quality Control Department when appropriate.

5.16. Access to production premises should be restricted to authorized personnel.

5.17. Normally, the production of non-medicinal products should be avoided in areas and with the equipment destined for the production of medicinal products.

Prevention of cross-contamination in production

5.18. Contamination of a starting material or of a product by another material or product must be avoided. This risk of accidental cross-contamination arises from the uncontrolled release of dust, gases, vapours, sprays or organisms from materials and products in process, from residues on equipment, and from operators' clothing. The significance of this risk varies with the type of contaminant and of product being contaminated. Amongst the most hazardous contaminants are highly sensitizing materials, biological preparations containing living organisms, certain hormones, cytotoxics, and other highly active materials. Products in which contamination is likely to be most significant are those administered by injection, those given in large doses and/or over a long time.

5.19. Cross-contamination should be avoided by appropriate technical or organisational measures, for example:

(a) production in segregated areas (required for products such as penicillins, live vaccines, live bacterial preparations and some other biologicals), or by campaign (separation in time) followed by appropriate cleaning;

(b) providing appropriate air-locks and air extraction;

(c) minimising the risk of contamination caused by recirculation or re-entry of untreated or insufficiently treated air;
(d) keeping protective clothing inside areas where products with special risk of cross-contamination are processed;
(e) using cleaning and decontamination procedures of known effectiveness, as ineffective cleaning of equipment is a common source of cross-contamination;
(f) using "closed systems" of production;
(g) testing for residues and use of cleaning status labels on equipment.

5.20. Measures to prevent cross-contamination and their effectiveness should be checked periodically according to set procedures.

Validation

5.21. Validation studies should reinforce Good Manufacturing Practice and be conducted in accordance with defined procedures. Results and conclusions should be recorded.

5.22. When any new manufacturing formula or method of preparation is adopted, steps should be taken to demonstrate its suitability for routine processing. The defined process, using the materials and equipment specified, should be shown to yield a product consistently of the required quality.

5.23. Significant amendments to the manufacturing process, including any change in equipment or materials, which may affect product quality and/or the reproducibility of the process should be validated.

5.24. Processes and procedures should undergo periodic critical re-validation to ensure that they remain capable of achieving the intended results.

Starting materials

5.25. The purchase of starting materials is an important operation which should involve staff who have a particular and thorough knowledge of the suppliers.

5.26. Starting materials should only be purchased from approved suppliers named in the relevant specification and, where possible, directly from the producer. It is recommended that the specifications established by the manufacturer for the starting materials be discussed with the suppliers. It is of benefit that all aspects of the production and control of the starting material in question, including handling, labelling and packaging requirements, as well as complaints and rejection procedures are discussed with the manufacturer and the supplier.

5.27. For each delivery, the containers should be checked for integrity of package and seal and for correspondence between the delivery note and the supplier's labels.

5.28. If one material delivery is made up of different batches, each batch must be considered as separate for sampling, testing and release.

5.29. Starting materials in the storage area should be appropriately labelled (see Chapter 5, Item 13). Labels should bear at least the following information:

- the designated name of the product and the internal code reference where applicable;
- a batch number given at receipt;
- where appropriate, the status of the contents (e.g. in quarantine, on test, released, rejected);
- where appropriate, an expiry date or a date beyond which retesting is necessary.

When fully computerized storage systems are used, all the above information need not necessarily be in a legible form on the label.

5.30. There should be appropriate procedures or measures to assure the identity of the contents of each container of starting material. Bulk containers from which samples have been drawn should be identified (see Chapter 6, Item 13).

5.31. Only starting materials which have been released by the Quality Control Department and which are within their shelf life should be used.

5.32. Starting materials should only be dispensed by designated persons, following a written procedure, to ensure that the correct materials are accurately weighed or measured into clean and properly labelled containers.

5.33. Each dispensed material and its weight or volume should be independently checked and the check recorded.

5.34. Materials dispensed for each batch should be kept together and conspicuously labelled as such.

Processing operations: intermediate and bulk products

5.35. Before any processing operation is started, steps should be taken to ensure that the work area and equipment are clean and free from any starting materials, products, product residues or documents not required for the current operation.

5.36. Intermediate and bulk products should be kept under appropriate conditions.

5.37. Critical processes should be validated (see "VALIDATION" in this Chapter).

5.38. Any necessary in-process controls and environmental controls should be carried out and recorded.

5.39. Any significant deviation from the expected yield should be recorded and investigated.

Packaging materials

5.40. The purchase, handling and control of primary and printed packaging materials shall be accorded attention similar to that given to starting materials.

5.41. Particular attention should be paid to printed materials. They should be stored in adequately secure conditions such as to exclude unauthorized access. Cut labels and other loose printed materials should be stored and transported in separate closed containers so as to avoid mix-ups. Packaging materials should be issued for use only by authorized personnel following an approved and documented procedure.

5.42. Each delivery or batch of printed or primary packaging material should be given a specific reference number or identification mark.

5.43. Outdated or obsolete primary packaging material or printed packaging material should be destroyed and this disposal recorded.

Packaging operations

5.44. When setting up a programme for the packaging operations, particular attention should be given to minimising the risk of cross-contamination, mix-ups or substitutions. Different products should not be packaged in close proximity unless there is physical segregation.

5.45. Before packaging operations are begun, steps should be taken to ensure that the work area, packaging lines, printing machines and other equipment are clean and free from any products, materials or documents previously used, if these are not required for the current operation. The line-clearance should be performed according to an appropriate check-list.

5.46. The name and batch number of the product being handled should be displayed at each packaging station or line.

5.47. All products and packaging materials to be used should be checked on delivery to the packaging department for quantity, identity and conformity with the Packaging Instructions.

5.48. Containers for filling should be clean before filling. Attention should be given to avoiding and removing any contaminants such as glass fragments and metal particles.

5.49. Normally, filling and sealing should be followed as quickly as possible by labelling. If it is not the case, appropriate procedures should be applied to ensure that no mix-ups or mislabelling can occur.

5.50. The correct performance of any printing operation (for example code numbers, expiry dates) to be done separately or in the course of the packaging should be checked and recorded. Attention should be paid to printing by hand which should be re-checked at regular intervals.

5.51. Special care should be taken when using cut-labels and when over-printing is carried out off-line. Roll-feed labels are normally preferable to cut-labels, in helping to avoid mix-ups.

5.52. Checks should be made to ensure that any electronic code readers, label counters or similar devices are operating correctly.

5.53. Printed and embossed information on packaging materials should be distinct and resistant to fading or erasing.

5.54. On-line control of the product during packaging should include at least checking the following:

(a) general appearance of the packages;
(b) whether the packages are complete;
(c) whether the correct products and packaging materials are used;
(d) whether any over-printing is correct;
(e) correct functioning of line monitors.

Samples taken away from the packaging line should not be returned.

5.55. Products which have been involved in an unusual event should only be reintroduced into the process after special inspection, investigation and approval by authorized personnel. Detailed record should be kept of this operation.

5.56. Any significant or unusual discrepancy observed during reconciliation of the amount of bulk product and printed packaging materials and the number of units produced should be investigated and satisfactorily accounted for before release.

5.57. Upon completion of a packaging operation, any unused batch-coded packaging materials should be destroyed and the destruction recorded. A documented procedure should be followed if uncoded printed materials are returned to stock.

Finished products

5.58. Finished products should be held in quarantine until their final release under conditions established by the manufacturer.

5.59. The evaluation of finished products and documentation which is necessary before release of product for sale are described in Chapter 6 (Quality Control).

5.60. After release, finished products should be stored as usable stock under conditions established by the manufacturer.

Rejected, recovered and returned materials

5.61. Rejected materials and products should be clearly marked as such and stored separately in restricted areas. They should either be returned to the suppliers or, where appropriate, reprocessed or destroyed. Whatever action is taken should be approved and recorded by authorized personnel.

5.62. The reprocessing of rejected products should be exceptional. It is only permitted if the quality of the final product is not affected, if the specifications are met and if it is done in accordance with a defined and authorized procedure after evaluation of the risks involved. Record should be kept of the reprocessing.

5.63. The recovery of all or part of earlier batches which conform to the required quality by incorporation into a batch of the same product at a defined stage of manufacture should be authorized beforehand. This recovery should be carried out in accordance with a defined procedure after evaluation of the risks involved, including any possible effect on shelf life. The recovery should be recorded.

5.64. The need for additional testing of any finished product which has been reprocessed, or into which a recovered product has been incorporated, should be considered by the Quality Control Department.

5.65. Products returned from the market and which have left the control of the manufacturer should be destroyed unless without doubt their quality is satisfactory; they may be considered for re-sale, re-labelling or recovery in a subsequent batch only after they have been critically assessed by the Quality Control Department in accordance with a written procedure. The nature of the product, any special storage conditions it requires, its condition and history, and the time elapsed since it was issued should all be taken into account in this assessment. Where any doubt arises over the quality of the product, it should not be considered suitable for re-issue or re-use, although basic chemical re-processing to recover active ingredient may be possible. Any action taken should be appropriately recorded.

6 QUALITY CONTROL

Principle

Quality Control is concerned with sampling, specifications and testing as well as the organisation, documentation and release procedures which ensure that the necessary and relevant tests are carried out, and that materials are not released for use, nor products released for sale or supply, until their quality has been judged satisfactory. Quality Control is not confined to laboratory operations, but must be involved in all decisions which may concern the quality of the product. The independence of Quality Control from Production is considered fundamental to the satisfactory operation of Quality Control. (see also Chapter 1).

General

6.1. Each holder of a manufacturing authorization should have a Quality Control Department. This department should be independent from other departments, and under the authority of a person with appropriate qualifications and experience, who has one or several control laboratories at his disposal. Adequate resources must be available to ensure that all the Quality Control arrangements are effectively and reliably carried out.

6.2. The principal duties of the head of Quality Control are summarized in Chapter 2. The Quality Control Department as a whole will also have other duties, such as to establish, validate and implement all quality control procedures, keep the reference samples of materials and products, ensure the correct labelling of containers of materials and products, ensure the monitoring of the stability of the products, participate in the investigation of complaints related to the quality of the product, etc. All these operations should be carried out in accordance with written procedures and, where necessary, recorded.

6.3. Finished product assessment should embrace all relevant factors, including production conditions, results of in-process testing, a review of manufacturing (including packaging) documentation, compliance with Finished Product Specification and examination of the final finished pack.

6.4. Quality Control personnel should have access to production areas for sampling and investigation as appropriate.

Good Quality Control Laboratory Practice

6.5 Control laboratory premises and equipment should meet the general and specific requirements for Quality Control areas given in Chapter 3.

6.6. The personnel, premises, and equipment in the laboratories should be appropriate to the tasks imposed by the nature and the scale of the manufacturing operations. The use of outside laboratories, in conformity with the principles detailed in Chapter 7, Contract Analysis, can be accepted for particular reasons, but this should be stated in the Quality Control records.

Documentation

6.7. Laboratory documentation should follow the principles given in Chapter 4. An important part of this documentation deals with Quality Control and the following details should be readily available to the Quality Control Department:

- specifications;
- sampling procedures;
- testing procedures and records (including analytical worksheets and/or laboratory notebooks);
- analytical reports and/or certificates;
- data from environmental monitoring, where required;
- validation records of test methods, where applicable;
- procedures for and records of the calibration of instruments and maintenance of equipment.

6.8. Any Quality Control documentation relating to a batch record should be retained for one year after the expiry date of the batch and at least 5 years after the certification referred to in article 22.2 of Directive 75/319/EEC.

6.9. For some kinds of data (e.g. analytical tests results, yields, environmental controls,...) it is recommended that records be kept in a manner permitting trend evaluation.

6.10. In addition to the information which is part of the batch record, other original data such as laboratory notebooks and/or records should be retained and readily available.

Sampling

6.11. The sample taking should be done in accordance with approved written procedures that describe:

- the method of sampling;
- the equipment to be used;
- the amount of the sample to be taken;
- instructions for any required sub-division of the sample;
- the type and condition of the sample container to be used;
- the identification of containers sampled;
- any special precautions to be observed, especially with regard to the sampling of sterile or noxious materials;

- the storage conditions;
- instructions for the cleaning and storage of sampling equipment.

6.12 Reference samples should be representative of the batch of materials or products from which they are taken. Other samples may also be taken to monitor the most stressed part of a process (e.g. beginning or end of a process).

6.13. Sample containers should bear a label indicating the contents, with the batch number, the date of sampling and the containers from which samples have been drawn.

6.14. Reference samples from each batch of finished products should be retained till one year after the expiry date. Finished products should usually be kept in their final packaging and stored under the recommended conditions. Samples of starting materials (other than solvents, gases and water) should be retained for at least two years(*) after the release of the product if their stability allows. This period may be shortened if their stability, as mentioned in the relevant specification, is shorter. Reference samples of materials and products should be of a size sufficient to permit at least a full re-examination.

Testing

6.15. Analytical methods should be validated. All testing operations described in the marketing authorization should be carried out according to the approved methods.

6.16. The results obtained should be recorded and checked to make sure that they are consistent with each other. Any calculations should be critically examined.

6.17. The tests performed should be recorded and the records should include at least the following data:

(a) name of the material or product and, where applicable, dosage form;
(b) batch number and, where appropriate, the manufacturer and/or supplier;
(c) references to the relevant specifications and testing procedures;
(d) test results, including observations and calculations, and reference to any certificates of analysis;
(e) dates of testing;
(f) initials of the persons who performed the testing;
(g) initials of the persons who verified the testing and the calculations, where appropriate;
(h) a clear statement of release or rejection (or other status decision) and the dated signature of the designated responsible person.

6.18. All the in-process controls, including those made in the production area by production personnel, should be performed according to methods approved by Quality Control and the results recorded.

(*) In Federal Republic of Germany, France, Belgium and Greece, samples of starting materials should be retained for as long as the corresponding finished product.

6.19. Special attention should be given to the quality of laboratory reagents, volumetric glassware and solutions, reference standards and culture media. They should be prepared in accordance with written procedures.

6.20. Laboratory reagents intended for prolonged use should be marked with the preparation date and the signature of the person who prepared them. The expiry date of unstable reagents and culture media should be indicated on the label, together with specific storage conditions. In addition, for volumetric solutions, the last date of standardisation and the last current factor should be indicated.

6.21. Where necessary, the date of receipt of any substance used for testing operations (e.g. reagents and reference standards) should be indicated on the container. Instructions for use and storage should be followed. In certain cases it may be necessary to carry out an identification test and/or other testing of reagent materials upon receipt or before use.

6.22. Animals used for testing components, materials or products, should, where appropriate, be quarantined before use. They should be maintained and controlled in a manner that assures their suitability for the intended use. They should be identified, and adequate records should be maintained, showing the history of their use.

7 CONTRACT MANUFACTURE AND ANALYSIS

Principle

Contract manufacture and analysis must be correctly defined, agreed and controlled in order to avoid misunderstandings which could result in a product or work of unsatisfactory quality. There must be a written contract between the Contract Giver and the Contract Acceptor which clearly establishes the duties of each party. The contract must clearly state the way in which the Qualified Person releasing each batch of product for sale exercises his full responsibility.

Note:

This Chapter deals with the responsibilities of manufacturers towards the Competent Authorities of the Member States with respect to the granting of marketing and manufacturing authorizations. It is not intended in any way to affect the respective liability of contract acceptors and contract givers to consumers; this is governed by other provisions of Community and national law.

General

7.1. There should be a written contract covering the manufacture and/or analysis arranged under contract and any technical arrangements made in connection with it.

7.2. All arrangements for contract manufacture and analysis including any proposed changes in technical or other arrangements should be in accordance with the marketing authorization for the product concerned.

The Contract Giver

7.3. The Contract Giver is responsible for assessing the competence of the Contract Acceptor to carry out successfully the work required and for ensuring by means of the contract that the principles and guidelines of GMP as interpreted in this Guide are followed.

7.4. The Contract Giver should provide the Contract Acceptor with all the information necessary to carry out the contracted operations correctly in accordance with the marketing authorisation and any other legal requirements. The Contract Giver should ensure that the Contract Acceptor is fully aware of any problems associated with the product or the work which might pose a hazard to his premises, equipment, personnel, other materials or other products.

7.5. The Contract Giver should ensure that all processed products and materials delivered to him by the Contract Acceptor comply with their specifications or that the products have been released by a Qualified Person.

The Contract Acceptor

7.6. The Contract Acceptor must have adequate premises and equipment, knowledge and experience, and competent personnel to carry out satisfactorily the work ordered by the Contract Giver. Contract manufacture may be undertaken only by a manufacturer who is the holder of a manufacturing authorization.

7.7. The Contract Acceptor should ensure that all products or materials delivered to him are suitable for their intended purpose.

7.8. The Contract Acceptor should not pass to a third party any of the work entrusted to him under the contract without the Contract Giver's prior evaluation and approval of the arrangements. Arrangements made between the Contract Acceptor and any third party should ensure that the manufacturing and analytical information is made available in the same way as between the original Contract Giver and Contract Acceptor.

7.9. The Contract Acceptor should refrain from any activity which may adversely affect the quality of the product manufactured and/or analysed for the Contract Giver.

The Contract

7.10. A contract should be drawn up between the Contract Giver and the Contract Acceptor which specifies their respective responsibilities relating to the manufacture and control of the product. Technical aspects of the contract should be drawn up by competent persons suitably knowledgeable in pharmaceutical technology, analysis and Good Manufacturing Practice. All arrangements for manufacture and analysis must be in accordance with the marketing authorisation and agreed by both parties.

7.11. The contract should specify the way in which the Qualified Person releasing the batch for sale ensures that each batch has been manufactured and checked for compliance with the requirements of Marketing Authorisation.

7.12. The contract should describe clearly who is responsible for purchasing materials, testing and releasing materials, undertaking production and quality controls, including in-process controls, and who has responsibility for sampling and analysis. In the case of contract analysis, the contract should state whether or not the Contract Acceptor should take samples at the premises of the manufacturer.

7.13. Manufacturing, analytical and distribution records, and reference samples should be kept by, or be available to, the Contract Giver. Any records relevant to assessing the quality of a product in the event of complaints or a suspected defect must be accessible and specified in the defect/recall procedures of the Contract Giver.

7.14. The contract should permit the Contract Giver to visit the facilities of the Contract Acceptor.

7.15. In the case of contract analysis, the Contract Acceptor should understand that he is subject to Inspection by the competent Authorities.

8 COMPLAINTS AND PRODUCT RECALL

Principle

All complaints and other information concerning potentially defective products must be reviewed carefully according to written procedures. In order to provide for all contingencies, and in accordance with Article 28 of Directive 75/319/EEC, a system should be designed to recall, if necessary, promptly and effectively products known or suspected to be defective from the market.

Complaints

8.1. A person should be designated responsible for handling the complaints and deciding the measures to be taken together with sufficient supporting staff to assist him. If this person is not the Qualified Person, the latter should be made aware of any complaint, investigation or recall.

8.2. There should be written procedures describing the action to be taken, including the need to consider a recall, in the case of a complaint concerning a possible product defect.

8.3. Any complaint concerning a product defect should be recorded with all the original details and thoroughly investigated. The person responsible for Quality Control should normally be involved in the study of such problems.

8.4. If a product defect is discovered or suspected in a batch, consideration should be given to checking other batches in order to determine whether they are also affected. In particular, other batches which may contain reworks of the defective batch should be investigated.

8.5. All the decisions and measures taken as a result of a complaint should be recorded and referenced to the corresponding batch records.

8.6. Complaints records should be reviewed regularly for any indication of specific or recurring problems requiring attention and possibly the recall of marketed products.

8.7. The Competent Authorities should be informed if a manufacturer is considering action following possibly faulty manufacture, product deterioration, or any other serious quality problems with a product.

Recalls

8.8. A person should be designated as responsible for execution and coordination of recalls and should be supported by sufficient staff to handle all the aspects of the recalls with the appropriate degree of urgency. This responsible person should normally be independent of the sales and marketing organization. If this person is not the Qualified Person, the latter should be made aware of any recall operation

8.9. There should be established written procedures, regularly checked and updated when necessary, in order to organize any recall activity.

8.10. Recall operations should be capable of being initiated promptly and at any time.

8.11 All Competent Authorities of all countries to which products may have been distributed should be informed promptly if products are intended to be recalled because they are, or are suspected of being defective.

8.12. The distribution records should be readily available to the person(s) responsible for recalls, and should contain sufficient information on wholesalers and directly supplied customers (with addresses, phone and/or fax numbers inside and outside working hours, batches and amounts delivered), including those for exported products and medical samples.

8.13. Recall products should be identified and stored separately in a secure area while awaiting a decision on their fate.

8.14. The progress of the recall process should be recorded and a final report issued, including a reconciliation between the delivered and recovered quantities of the products.

8.15 The effectiveness of the arrangements for recalls should be evaluated from time to time.

9 SELF INSPECTION

Principle

Self inspections should be conducted in order to monitor the implementation and compliance with Good Manufacturing Practice principles and to propose necessary corrective measures.

9.1. Personnel matters, premises, equipment, documentation, production, quality control, distribution of the medicinal products, arrangements for dealing with complaints and recalls, and self inspection, should be examined at intervals following a pre-arranged programme in order to verify their conformity with the principles of Quality Assurance.

9.2. Self inspections should be conducted in an independent and detailed way by designated competent person(s) form the company. Independent audits by external experts may also be useful.

9.3. All self inspections should be recorded. Reports should contain all the observations made during the inspections and, where applicable, proposals for corrective measures. Statements on the actions subsequently taken should also be recorded.

Annexes

ANNEX 1 MANUFACTURE OF STERILE MEDICINAL PRODUCTS

Principle

The manufacture of sterile preparations has special requirements in order to minimize risks of microbiological contamination, and of particulate and pyrogen contamination. Much depends on the skill, training and attitudes of the personnel involved. Quality Assurance bears a particularly great importance, and this manufacture must strictly follow carefully established and validated methods of preparation and procedures.

General

1. Production of sterile preparations should be carried out in clean areas whose entry should be through airlocks for personnel or for goods. Clean areas should be maintained to an appropriate cleanliness standard and supplied with air which has all passed through filters of an appropriate efficiency.

2. The various operations of component preparation, product preparation, filling and sterilisation should be carried out in separate areas within the clean area.

3. Clean areas for production of sterile products are classified according to the required characteristics of the air, in grades A, B, C and D. The air characteristics are given in the table below.

Air classification system for manufacture of sterile products

Grade	Max. permitted number of particles per m3 equal to or above:		Max. permitted No. of viable micro-organisms per m^3
	0.5µm	5µm	
A Laminar air flow work station	3,500	none	less than 1*
B	3,500	none	5*
C	350,000	2,000	100
D	3,500,000	20,000	500

Notes:

– Laminar air flow systems should provide an homogeneous air speed of 0.30 m/s for vertical flow and 0.45 m/s for horizontal flow.

- In order to reach the B, C and D air grades, the number of air changes should generally be higher than 20 per hour in a room with a good air flow pattern and appropriate HEPA filters.

- Low values involved here* are only reliable when a large number of air samples are taken.

- The guidance given for the maximum permitted number of particles corresponds approximately to the US Federal Standard 209 C as follows: Class 100 (grades A and B), Class 10 000 (grade C) and Class 100 000 (grade D).

- It is accepted that it may not always be possible to demonstrate conformity with particulate standards at the point of fill when filling is in progress, due to generation of particles or droplets from the product itself.

4. Each manufacturing operation requires an appropriate air cleanliness level in order to minimize the risks of particulate or microbial contamination of the product or materials being handled. Items 5 and 6 give the minimum air-grades required for different manufacturing operations. The particulate and microbiological conditions given in the table should be maintained in the zone immediately surrounding the product whenever the product is exposed to the environment. The conditions should be achieved throughout the background environment where unmanned, and recovered after a short "clean up" period.

   The utilisation of absolute barrier technology and automated systems to minimize human interventions in processing areas can produce significant advantages in assurance of sterility of manufactured products. When such techniques are used, the recommendations in these Supplementary Guidelines, particularly those relating to air quality and monitoring, still apply, with appropriate interpretation of the terms "work station" and "environment".

   Manufacturing operations are here divided into two categories, first those where the preparation is terminally sterilized, sealed in its final container, and second those which must be conducted in an aseptic way at some or all stages.

Terminally sterilized products

5. Preparation of solutions should be done in a grade C environment in order to give low microbial and particulate counts, suitable for filtration and sterilisation. It could be allowed in a grade D environment, provided additional steps are taken in order to minimize the contamination, such as the use of closed vessels.

   Filling large volume parenterals should be done under a laminar air flow work station, in a grade C environment. The same conditions are recommended for small volume parenterals.

   Preparation and filling of ointments, creams, suspensions and emulsions should generally be done in a grade C environment before terminal sterilization.

Aseptic preparations

6. Handling of starting materials should be done in a grade C environment, if sterile filtered later in the process; if not, in a grade A zone with a grade B background.

   Preparation of solutions which are to be sterile filtered during the process should be done in a grade C environment; if not filtered, it should be done in a grade A environment with a grade B background.

   Handling and filling of aseptically prepared products including small and large volume parenterals, should be done in a grade A environment, with a grade B background.

   Preparation and filling of ointments, creams, suspensions and emulsions should be done in a grade A environment, background of grade B, when the product is exposed and is not subsequently filtered.

Personnel

7. Only the minimum number of personnel required should be present in clean areas; this is particularly important in during aseptic processes. Inspections and controls should be conducted from outside the areas as far as possible.

8. All personnel (including those concerned with cleaning and maintenance) employed in such areas should receive regular training in disciplines relevant to the correct manufacture of sterile products, including reference to hygiene and to the basic elements of microbiology. When outside staff who have not received such training (e.g. building or maintenance contractors) need to be brought in, particular care should be taken over their supervision.

9. Staff who have been engaged in the processing of animal tissue materials or of cultures of micro-organisms other than those used in the current manufacturing process should not enter sterile-product areas unless rigorous and clearly defined decontamination procedures have been followed.

10. High standards of personal hygiene and cleanliness are essential, and personnel involved in the manufacture of sterile preparations should be instructed to report any condition which may cause the shedding of abnormal numbers or types of contaminants; periodic health checks for such conditions are desirable. Actions to be taken about personnel who could be introducing undue microbiological hazard should be decided by a designated competent person.

11. Outdoor clothing should not be brought into the clean areas, and personnel entering the changing rooms should already be clad in standard factory protective garments. Changing and washing should follow a written procedure.

12. The clothing and its quality should be appropriate for the process and the working area, and worn in such a way as to protect the product from contamination.

13. Wristwatches and jewellery should not be worn in clean areas and cosmetics which can shed particles should not be used.

14. Clothing should be appropriate for the air grade of the area where the personnel will be working. The description of clothing required for each grade is given below:

    Grade D: Hair and, where appropriate, beard should be covered. A general protective clothing and appropriate shoes or overshoes should be worn. Appropriate measures should be taken to avoid any contamination coming from outside the clean area.

    Grade C: Hair and, where appropriate, beard should be covered. A single or two-piece trouser suit, gathered at the wrists and with high neck and appropriate shoes or overshoes should be worn. They should shed virtually no fibres or particulate matter.

    Grade B: A headgear should totally enclose hair and, where appropriate, beard; it should be tucked into the neck of the suit; a face mask should be worn to prevent the shedding of droplets; sterilized non powdered rubber or plastic gloves and sterilised or disinfected footwear should be worn; trouser-bottoms should be tucked inside the footwear as well as garment sleeves into the gloves. The protective clothing should shed virtually no fibres or particulate matter and retain particles shed by the body.

15. For every worker in a grade B room, clean sterilised protective garments should be provided at each work session, or at least once a day if monitoring results justify this. Gloves should be regularly disinfected during operations and masks and gloves should be changed at least at every working session. The use of disposable clothing may be necessary in certain circumstances.

16. Clean area clothing should be laundered or cleaned in such a way that it does not gather additional particulate contaminants which can later be shed. Separate laundry facilities for such clothing are desirable. Damaging fibers by inappropriate cleaning or sterilization may increase the risk of shedding of particles. Washing and sterilisation operations should follow written procedures.

Premises

17. In clean areas, all exposed surfaces should be smooth, impervious and unbroken in order to minimize the shedding or accumulation of particles or microorganisms and to permit the repeated application of cleaning agents, and disinfectants where used.

18. To reduce accumulation of dust and to facilitate cleaning there should be no uncleanable recesses and a minimum of projecting ledges, shelves, cupboards and equipment. Doors should be carefully designed to avoid those uncleanable recesses; sliding doors are undesirable for this reason.

19. False ceilings should be sealed to prevent contamination from the space above them.

20. Pipes and ducts should be installed so that they do not create recesses which are difficult to clean.

21. Sinks and drains should be avoided wherever possible and should be excluded from areas where aseptic operations are done. Where installed they should be designed, located and maintained so as to minimise risks of microbial contamination; they should be fitted with effective, easily cleanable traps and with air breaks to prevent back-flow. Any floor channel should be open, shallow and easily cleanable and be connected to drains outside the area in a manner which prevents ingress of microbial contaminants.

22. Changing rooms should be designed as airlocks and used to provide separation of the different stages of changing and so minimize microbial and particulate contamination of protective clothing. They should be effectively flushed with filtered air. The use of separate changing rooms for entering and leaving clean areas is sometimes desired. Hand washing facilities should be provided only in the changing rooms.

23. Airlock doors should not be opened simultaneously. An interlocking system or a visual and/or audible warning system should be operated to prevent the opening of more than one door.

24. A filtered air supply should maintain a positive pressure relative to surrounding areas under all operational conditions and should flush the area effectively. Particular attention should be paid to the protection of the zone of greatest risk, that is, the immediate environment to which a product and cleaned components which contact the product are exposed. The various recommendations regarding air supplies and pressure differentials may need to be modified where it becomes necessary to contain some materials, e.g. pathogenic, highly toxic, radioactive or live viral or bacterial materials or products. Decontamination facilities and treatment of air leaving a clean area may be necessary for some operations.

25. It should be demonstrated that air-flow patterns do not present a contamination risk, e.g. care should be taken to ensure that air-flows do not distribute particles from a particles-generating person, operation, or machine to a zone of higher product risk.

26. A warning system should be provided to indicate failure in the air supply. Indicators of pressure differences should be fitted between areas where these differences are important. These pressure differences should be recorded regularly.

Equipment

27. A conveyor belt should not pass through a partition between a clean area B and a processing area of lower air cleanliness, unless the belt itself is continually sterilised (e.g. in a sterilising tunnel).

28. As far as possible equipment fittings and services should be designed and installed so that operations, maintenance and repairs can be carried out outside the clean area. If sterilisation is required, it should be carried out after complete reassembly wherever possible.

29. When equipment maintenance has been carried out within the clean area, the area should be cleaned, and disinfected where appropriate, before processing recommences if the required standards of cleanliness and/or asepsis have not been maintained during the work.

30. All equipment including sterilizers, air filtration systems, water treatment systems including stills should be subject to planned maintenance and validation; their use following maintenance work should be approved by the Quality Control.

31. Water treatment plants should be designed, constructed and maintained so as to ensure the reliable production of water of an appropriate quality. They should not be operated beyond their designed capacity. Water should be produced, stored and distributed in a manner which prevents microbial growth, for example by constant circulation at a temperature above 70°C.

Sanitation

32. The sanitation of clean areas is particularly important They should be cleaned frequently and thoroughly in accordance with a written programme approved by the Quality Control department. Where disinfectants are used, more than one type should be employed. Monitoring should be undertaken regularly in order to detect the development of resistant strains.

33. Disinfectants and detergents should be monitored for microbial contamination; dilutions should be kept in previously cleaned containers and should not be stored for long periods unless sterilised. Partly emptied containers should not be topped up.

34. Fumigation of clean areas may be useful for reducing microbiological contamination in inaccessible places.

35. Clean areas should be monitored at planned intervals during operations by means of microbial counts; where aseptic operations are performed, monitoring should be frequent and the results considered when determining batch approval. Additional monitoring is sometimes also desirable outside production operations, e.g. after validation of systems, cleaning, fumigation.

Processing

36. Precautions to minimize contamination should be taken during all processing stages including the stages before sterilisation.

37. Preparations of microbiological origin should not be made or filled in areas used for the processing of other medicinal products; however, vaccines of dead organisms or of bacterial extracts may be filled, after inactivation, in the same premises as other sterile medicinal products.

38. Aseptic processes or significant modifications should be validated by using a sterile nutrient medium for simulating the process to be performed. That validation should be repeated at defined intervals.

39. Care should be taken that validations do not hazard the processes.

40. Water sources, water treatment equipment and treated water should be monitored regularly for chemical and biological contamination and, as appropriate, for endotoxins. Records should be maintained of the results of the monitoring and of any action taken.

41. Activities in clean areas and especially when aseptic operations are in progress should be kept to a minimum and movement of personnel should be controlled and methodical, to avoid excessive shedding of particles and organisms due to over-vigorous activity. The ambient temperature and humidity should not be uncomfortably high because of the nature of the garments worn.

42. Microbiological contamination of starting materials should be minimal. The bioburden should be monitored before sterilisation. Specifications should include requirements for microbiological quality when the need for this has been indicated by monitoring.

43. Containers and materials liable to generate fibres should be minimized in clean areas and avoided completely when aseptic work is in progress.

44. Components, containers and equipment should be handled after the final cleaning process in such a way that they are not recontaminated.

45. The interval between the washing and drying and the sterilisation of components, containers and equipment as well as between their sterilisation and use should be as short as possible and subject to a time-limit appropriate to the storage conditions.

46. The time between the start of the preparation of a solution and its sterilisation or filtration through a bacteria-retaining filter should be as short as possible. There should be a set maximum permissible time for each product that takes into account its composition and the prescribed method of storage.

47. The microbiological contamination of products should be minimal prior to sterilisation. There should be a working limit on contamination immediately before sterilisation which is related to the efficiency of the method to be used and the risk of pyrogens. All solutions, in particular large volume infusion fluids, should be passed through a micro-organisms retaining filter, if possible immediately before filling.

48. Components, containers, equipment and any other article required in a clean area where aseptic work is in progress should be sterilised and passed into the area through double-ended sterilisers sealed into the wall, or by a procedure which achieves the same end of not introducing contamination.

49. The efficacy of any new procedure should be validated, and the validation repeated at regular intervals thereafter, or, when any significant change is made in the process or equipment.

Sterilisation

50. All sterilisation processes should be validated. Particular attention should be given when the adopted sterilisation method is not described in the current edition of the European Pharmacopoeia, or when it is used for a preparation which is not a simple aqueous or oily solution. Where possible and practicable, heat sterilisation is the method of choice. In any case, the sterilisation process must be in accordance with the marketing and manufacturing authorizations.

51. Before any sterilisation process is adopted its suitability for the product and its efficacy in achieving the desired sterilising conditions in all parts of each type of load to be processed should be demonstrated. This work should be repeated at scheduled intervals, at least annually, and whenever significant modifications have been made to the equipment. Records should be kept of the results.

52. For effective sterilisation the whole of the material must be subjected to the required treatment and the process should be designed to ensure that this is achieved.

53. Biological indicators should be considered only as an additional method for monitoring the sterilisation. If they are used, strict precautions should be taken to avoid transferring microbial contamination from them.

54. There should be a clear means of differentiating products which have not been sterilised from those which have. Each basket, tray or other carrier of products or components should be clearly labelled with the material name, its batch number and an indication of whether or not it has been sterilised. Indicators such as autoclave tape may be used, where appropriate, to indicate whether or not a batch (or sub-batch) has passed through a sterilisation process, but they do not give a reliable indication that the lot is, in fact, sterile.

Sterilisation by heat

55. Each heat sterilisation cycle should be recorded on a time/temperature chart with a suitably large scale or by other appropriate equipment with suitable accuracy and precision. The temperature should be recorded from a probe at the coolest part of the load or loaded chamber, this point having been determined during the validation, and preferably also checked against a second independent temperature probe located at the same position. The Chart, or a photocopy thereof, should form part of the batch record. Chemical or biological indicators may also be used, but should not take the place of physical controls.

56. Sufficient time must be allowed for the whole of the load to reach the required temperature before measurement of the sterilising time-period is commenced. This time must be determined for each type of load to be processed.

57. After the high temperature phase of a heat sterilisation cycle, precautions should be taken against contamination of a sterilised load during cooling. Any cooling fluid or gas in contact with the product should be sterilized, unless it can be shown that any leaking container would not be approved for use.

Moist heat

58. Both temperature and pressure should be used to monitor the process. The temperature recorder should normally be independent of the controller, and there should be an independent temperature indicator, the reading from which is routinely checked against the chart recorder during the sterilisation period. For sterilisers fitted with a drain at the bottom of the chamber, it may also be necessary to record the temperature at this position, throughout the sterilisation period. There should be frequent leak tests on the chamber when a vacuum phase is part of the cycle.

59. The items to be sterilised, other than products in sealed containers, should be wrapped in a material which allows removal of air and penetration of steam but which prevents recontamination after sterilisation. All parts of the load should be in contact with water or saturated steam at the required temperature for the required time.

60. Care should be taken to ensure that steam used for sterilisation is of suitable quality and does not contain additives at a level which could cause contamination of product or equipment.

Dry heat

61. The process used should include air circulation within the chamber and the maintenance of a positive pressure to prevent the entry of non-sterile air. Any air admitted should be passed through a micro-organisms retaining filter. Where this process is also intended to remove pyrogens, challenge tests using endotoxins may be required as part of the validation.

Sterilisation by radiation

62. Radiation sterilisation is used mainly for the sterilisation of heat sensitive materials and products. Many medicinal products and some packaging materials are radiation-sensitive, so this method is permissible only when the absence of deleterious effects on the product has been confirmed experimentally. Ultraviolet irradiation is not normally an acceptable method of sterilisation.

63. During the sterilisation procedure the radiation dose should be measured. For this purpose, dosimetry indicators which are independent of dose rate should be used, giving a quantitative measurement of the dose received by the product itself. Dosimeters should be inserted in the load in sufficient number, and close enough together to ensure that there is always a dosimeter in the chamber. Where plastic dosimeters are used they should be used within the time-limit of their calibration. Dosimeter absorbances should be read within a short period after exposure to radiation.

    Biological indicators may only be used as an additional control. Radiation-sensitive colour disks may also be used to differentiate between packages which have been subjected to irradiation and those which have not; they are not indicators of successful sterilisation. The information obtained should constitute part of the batch record.

64. Validation procedures should ensure that the effects of variations in density of the packages are considered.

65. Materials handling procedures should prevent mix-up between irradiated and non-irradiated materials. Each package should carry a radiation-sensitive indicator to show whether or not it has been subjected to a radiation treatment.

66. The total radiation dose should be administered within a predetermined timespan.

Sterilisation with ethylene oxide

67. This method should only be used when no other method is practicable. During process validation it should be shown that there is no damaging effect on the product and that the conditions and time allowed for degassing are such as to reduce any residual gas and reaction products to defined acceptable limits for the type of product or material.

68. Direct contact between gas and microbial cells is essential: precautions should be taken to avoid the presence of organisms likely to be enclosed in material such as crystals or dried protein. The nature and quantity of packaging materials can significantly affect the process.

69. Before exposure to the gas, materials should be brought into equilibrium with the humidity and temperature required by the process. The time required for this

should be balanced against the opposing need to minimise the time before sterilisation.

70. Each sterilisation cycle should be monitored with suitable biological indicators, using the appropriate number of test pieces distributed throughout the load. The information so obtained should form part of the batch record.

71. Biological indicators should be stored and used according to the manufacturers instructions, and their performance checked by positive controls.

72. For each sterilisation cycle, records should be made of the time taken to complete the cycle, of the pressure, temperature and humidity within the chamber during the process and of the gas concentration. The pressure and temperature should be recorded throughout the cycle on a chart. The record(s) should form part of the batch record.

73. After sterilisation, the load should be stored in a controlled manner under ventilated conditions to allow residual gas and reaction products to reduce to the defined level. This process should be validated.

Filtration of medicinal products which cannot be sterilised in their final container

74. Filtration alone is not considered sufficient when sterilisation in the final container is practicable. With regard to methods currently available, steam sterilisation is to be preferred. If the product cannot be sterilised in the final container, solutions or liquids can be filtered through a sterile filter of nominal pore size of 0.22 micron (or less), or with at least equivalent micro-organism retaining properties, into a previously sterilised container. Such filters can remove bacteria and moulds, but not all viruses or mycoplasmas. Consideration should be given to complementing the filtration process with some degree of heat treatment.

75. Due to the potential additional risks of the filtration method as compared with other sterilisation processes, a second filtration via a further sterilised micro-organism retaining filter, immediately prior to filling, may be advisable. The final sterile filtration should be carried out as close as possible to the filling point.

76. Fibres-shedding filters should not be used.

77. The integrity of the filter should be checked by an appropriate method such as a bubble point test immediately after each use (it may also be useful to test the filter in this way before use). The time taken to filter a known volume of bulk solution and the pressure difference to be used across the filter should be determined during validation and any significant differences from this should be noted and investigated. Results of these checks should be recorded in the batch record.

78. The same filter should not be used for more than one working day unless such use has been validated.

79. The filter should not affect the product by removal of ingredients from it or by release of substances into it.

Finishing of sterile products

80. Containers should be closed by appropriately validated methods. Samples should be checked for integrity according to appropriate procedures.

81. Containers sealed under vacuum should be sampled and the samples tested for maintenance of that vacuum after an appropriate, pre-determined period.

82. Filled containers of parenteral products should be inspected individually. When inspection is done visually, it should be done under suitable and controlled conditions of illumination and background. Operators doing the inspection should pass regular eye-sight checks, with spectacles if worn, and be allowed frequent breaks from inspection. Where other methods of inspection are used, the process should be validated and the performance of the equipment checked at intervals.

Quality Control

83. The sterility test applied to the finished product should only be regarded as the last in a series of control measures by which sterility is assured.

84. Samples taken for sterility testing should be representative of the whole of the batch, but should in particular include samples taken from parts of the batch considered to be most at risk of contamination, e.g.:
    (a) for products which have been filled aseptically, samples should include containers filled at the beginning and end of the batch and after any significant interruption of work;
    (b) for products which have been heat sterilised in their final containers, consideration should be given to taking samples from the potentially coolest part of the load.

85. For injectable products, consideration should be given to monitoring the water, the intermediate and the finished product for endotoxins, according to the European Pharmacopoeia method. The method should be validated for each type of product. For large volume infusion solutions such monitoring of water or intermediates should always be done in addition to any tests required by the marketing authorization on the finished product. When a sample fails the test, the cause of failure should be investigated and remedial action taken where necessary.

ANNEX 2 MANUFACTURE OF BIOLOGICAL MEDICINAL PRODUCTS FOR HUMAN USE

Scope:

The methods employed in the manufacture of biological medicinal products are a critical factor in shaping the appropriate regulatory control. Biological medicinal products can be defined therefore largely by reference to their method of manufacture. Biological medicinal products prepared by the following methods of manufacture will fall under the scope of this annex (1).

(a) Microbial cultures, excluding those resulting from r-DNA techniques;

(b) Microbial and cell cultures, including those resulting from recombinant DNA or hybridoma techniques;

(c) Extraction from biological tissues

(d) Propagation of live agents in embryos or animals

(Not all of the aspects of this annex may necessarily apply to products in category a).

Note:

In drawing up this guidance, due consideration has been given to the general requirements for manufacturing establishments and control laboratories proposed by the WHO.

The present guidance does not lay down detailed requirements for specific classes of biological products, and attention is therefore directed to other guidelines issued by the Committee for Proprietary Medicinal Products (CPMP), for example the note for guidance on monoclonal antibodies and the note for guidance on products of recombinant DNA technology ("The rules governing medicinal product in the European Community", Volume III).

Principle

The manufacture of biological medicinal products involves certain specific considerations arising from the nature of the products and the processes. The way in which biological medicinal products are produced, controlled and administered make some particular precautions necessary.

Unlike conventional medicinal products, which are reproduced using chemical and physical techniques capable of a high degree of consistency, the production of biological medicinal products involves biological processes and materials, such as cultivation of cells or extraction of material from living organisms. These biological processes may display

---

(1) Biological medicinal products manufactured by these methods include: vaccines, immunosera, antigens, hormones, cytokines, enzymes and other products of fermentation (including monoclonal antibodies and products derived from r-DNA).

inherent variability, so that the range and nature of by-products are variable. Moreover, the materials used in these cultivation processes provide good substrates for growth of microbial contaminants.

Control of biological medicinal products usually involves biological analytical techniques which have a greater variability than physico-chemical determinations. In-process controls therefore take on a great importance in the manufacture of biological medicinal products.

Personnel

1. All personnel (including those concerned with cleaning, maintenance or quality control) employed in areas where biological medicinal products are manufactured should receive additional training specific to the products manufactured and to their work. Personnel should be given relevant information and training in hygiene and microbiology.

2. Persons responsible for production and quality control should have an adequate background in relevant scientific disciplines, such as bacteriology, biology, biometry, chemistry, medicine, pharmacy, pharmacology, virology, immunology and veterinary medicine, together with sufficient practical experience to enable them to exercise their management function for the process concerned.

3. The immunological status of personnel may have to be taken into consideration for product safety. All personnel engaged in production, maintenance, testing and animal care (and inspectors) should be vaccinated where necessary with appropriate specific vaccines and have regular health checks. Apart from the obvious problem of exposure of staff to infectious agents, potent toxins or allergens, it is necessary to avoid the risk of contamination of a production batch with infectious agents. Visitors should generally be excluded from production areas.

4. Any changes in the immunological status of personnel which could adversely affect the quality of the product should preclude work in the production area. Production of BCG vaccine and tuberculin products should be restricted to staff who are carefully monitored by regular checks of immunological status or chest X-ray.

5. In the course of a working day, personnel should not pass from areas where exposure to live organisms or animals is possible to areas where other products or different organisms are handled. If such passage is unavoidable, clearly defined decontamination measures, including change of clothing and shoes and, where necessary, showering should be followed by staff involved in any such production.

Premises and Equipment

6. The degree of environmental control of particulate and microbial contamination of the production premises should be adapted to the product and the production step,

bearing in mind the level of contamination of the starting materials and the risk to the finished product.

7. The risk of cross-contamination between biological medicinal products, especially during those stages of the manufacturing process in which live organisms are used, may require additional precautions with respect to facilities and equipment, such as the use of dedicated facilities and equipment, production on a campaign basis and the use of closed systems. The nature of the product as well as the equipment used will determine the level of segregation needed to avoid cross-contamination.

8. In principle, dedicated facilities should be used for the production of BCG vaccine and for the handling of live organisms used in production of tuberculin products.

9. Dedicated facilities should be used for the handling of Bacillus anthracis, of Clostridium botulinum and of Clostridium tetani until the inactivation process is accomplished.

10. Production on a campaign basis may be acceptable for other spore forming organisms provided that the facilities are dedicated to this group of products and not more than one product is processed at any one time.

11. Simultaneous production in the same area using closed systems of biofermenters may be acceptable for products such as monoclonal antibodies and products prepared by rDNA techniques.

12. Processing steps after harvesting may be carried out simultaneously in the same production area provided that adequate precautions are taken to prevent cross contamination. For killed vaccines and toxoids, such parallel processing should only be performed after inactivation of the culture or after detoxification.

13. Positive pressure areas should be used to process sterile products but negative pressure in specific areas at point of exposure of pathogens is acceptable for containment reasons.

    Where negative pressure areas or safety cabinets are used for aseptic processing of pathogens, they should be surrounded by a positive pressure sterile zone.

14. Air filtration units should be specific to the processing area concerned and recirculation of air should not occur from areas handling live pathogenic organisms.

15. The layout and design of production areas and equipment should permit effective cleaning and decontamination (e.g. by fumigation). The adequacy of cleaning and decontamination procedures should be validated.

16. Equipment used during handling of live organisms should be designed to maintain cultures in a pure state and uncontaminated by external sources during processing.

17. Pipework systems, valves and vent filters should be properly designed to facilitate cleaning and sterilization. The use of 'clean in place' and 'sterilize in place' systems should be encouraged. Valves on fermentation vessels should be completely steam

sterilisable. Air vent filters should be hydrophobic and validated for their scheduled life span.

18. Primary containment should be designed and tested to demonstrate freedom from leakage risk.

19. Effluents which may contain pathogenic microorganisms should be effectively decontaminated.

20. Due to the variability of biological products or processes, some additives or ingredients have to be measured or weighed during the production process (e.g. buffers). In these cases, small stocks of these substances may be kept in the production area.

Animal quarters and care

21. Animals are used for the manufacture of a number of biological products, for example polio vaccine (monkeys), snake antivenoms (horses and goats), rabies vaccine (rabbits, mice and hamsters) and serum gonadotropin (horses). In addition, animals may also be used in the quality control of most sera and vaccines, e.g. pertussis vaccine (mice), pyrogenicity (rabbits), BCG vaccine (guinea-pigs).

22. General requirements for animal quarters, care and quarantine are laid down in Directive 86/609/EEC. Quarters for animals used in production and control of biological products should be separated from production and control areas. The health status of animals from which some starting materials are derived and of those used for quality control and safety testing should be monitored and recorded. Staff employed in such areas must be provided with special clothing and changing facilities. Where monkeys are used for the production or quality control of biological medicinal products, special consideration is required as laid down in the current WHO Requirements for Biological Substances no 7.

Documentation

23. Specifications for biological starting materials may need additional documentation on the source, origin, method of manufacture and controls applied, particularly microbiological controls.

24. Specifications are routinely required for intermediate and bulk biological medicinal products.

Production

Starting materials

25. The source, origin and suitability of starting materials should be clearly defined. Where the necessary tests take a long time, it may be permissible to process start-

ing materials before the results of the tests are available. In such cases, release of a finished product is conditional on satisfactory results of these tests.

26. Where sterilization of starting materials is required, it should be carried out where possible by heat. Where necessary, other appropriate methods may also be used for inactivation of biological materials (e.g. irradiation).

Seed lot and cell bank system.

27. In order to prevent the unwanted drift of properties which might ensue from repeated subcultures or multiple generations, the production of biological medicinal products obtained by microbial culture, cell culture or propagation in embryos and animals should be based on a system of master and working seed lots and/or cell banks.

28. The number of generations (doublings, passages) between the seed lot or cell bank and the finished product should be consistent with the marketing authorization dossier. Scaling up of the process should not change this fundamental relationship.

29. Seed lots and cell banks should be adequately characterized and tested for contaminants. Their suitability for use should be further demonstrated by the consistency of the characteristics and quality of the successive batches of product. Seed lots and cell banks should be established, stored and used in such a way as to minimize the risks of contamination or alteration.

30. Establishment of the seed lot and cell bank should be performed in a suitably controlled environment to protect the seed lot and the cell bank and, if applicable, the personnel handling it. During the establishment of the seed lot and cell bank, no other living or infectious material (e.g. virus, cell lines or cell strains) should be handled simultaneously in the same area or by the same persons.

31. Evidence of the stability and recovery of the seeds and banks should be documented. Storage containers should be hermetically sealed, clearly labelled and kept at an appropriate temperature. An inventory should be meticulously kept. Storage temperature should be recorded continuously for freezers and properly monitored for liquid nitrogen. Any deviation from set limits and any corrective action taken should be recorded.

32. Only authorized personnel should be allowed to handle the material and this handling should be done under the supervision of a responsible person. Access to stored material should be controlled. Different seed lots or cell banks should be stored in such a way to avoid confusion or cross-contamination. It is desirable to split the seed lots and cell banks and to store the parts at different locations so as to minimize the risks of total loss.

33. All containers of master or working cell banks and seed lots should be treated identically during storage. Once removed from storage, the containers should not be returned to the stock.

Operating principles

34. The growth promoting properties of culture media should be demonstrated.

35. Addition of materials or cultures to fermenters and other vessels and the taking of samples should be carried out under carefully controlled conditions to ensure that absence of contamination is maintained. Care should be taken to ensure that vessels are correctly connected when addition or sampling take place.

36. Centrifugation and blending of products can lead to aerosol formation and containment of such activities to prevent transfer of live microorganisms is necessary.

37. If possible, media should be sterilized in situ. In-line sterilizing filters for routine addition of gases, media, acids or alkalis, defoaming agents etc. to fermenters should be used where possible.

38. Careful consideration should be given to the validation of any necessary virus removal or inactivation undertaken (see CPMP notes for guidance).

39. In cases where a virus inactivation or removal process is performed during manufacture, measures should be taken to avoid the risk of recontamination of treated products by non-treated products.

40. A wide variety of equipment is used for chromatography, and in general such equipment should be dedicated to the purification of one product and should be sterilized or sanitized between batches. The use of the same equipment at different stages of processing should be discouraged. Acceptance criteria, life span and sanitization or sterilization method of columns should be defined.

Quality control

41. In-process controls play a specially important role in ensuring the consistency of the quality of biological medicinal products. Those controls which are crucial for quality (e.g. virus removal) but which cannot be carried out on the finished product, should be performed at an appropriate stage of production.

42. It may be necessary to retain samples of intermediate products in sufficient quantities and under appropriate storage conditions to allow the repetition or confirmation of a batch control.

43. Continuous monitoring of certain production processes is necessary, for example fermentation. Such data should form part of the batch record.

44. Where continuous culture is used, special consideration should be given to the quality control requirements arising from this type of production method.

ANNEX 3 MANUFACTURE OF RADIOPHARMACEUTICALS

Principle

The manufacturing and handling of radiopharmaceuticals is potentially hazardous. The level of risk depends in particular upon the types of radiation emitted and the half-lives of the radioactive isotopes. Particular attention must be paid to the prevention of cross-contamination, to the retention of radionuclide contaminants, and to waste disposal. Special consideration may be necessary with reference to the small batch sizes made frequently for many radiopharmaceuticals. Due to their short half-life, some radiopharmaceuticals are released before completion of certain Quality Control tests. In this case, the continuous assessment of the effectiveness of the Quality Assurance system becomes very important.

Note

Manufacture must comply with the requirements of EURATOM Directives laying down the basic standards for the health protection of the general public and workers against the dangers of ionizing radiation, as well as complying with other relevant national requirements.

Personnel

1. All personnel (including those concerned with cleaning and maintenance) employed in areas where radioactive products are manufactured should receive additional training specific to this class of products. In particular, they should be given detailed information and appropriate training on radiation protection.

Premises and equipment

2. Radioactive products should be stored, processed, packaged and controlled in dedicated and self-contained facilities. The equipment used for manufacturing operations should be reserved exclusively for radiopharmaceuticals.

3. In order to contain the radioactive particles, it may be necessary for the air pressure to be lower where products are exposed than in surrounding areas. However, it is still necessary to protect the product from environmental contamination.

4. For sterile products the working zone where products or containers may be exposed should comply with the environmental requirements described in the Supplement on Sterile Products. This may be achieved by the provision within the work station of a laminar flow of HEPA-filtered air and by fitting air-locks to entry

ports. Total containment work stations may provide these requirements. They should be in an environment conforming to at least grade D.

5. Air extracted from areas where radioactive products are handled should not be recirculated; air outlets should be designed to avoid possible environmental contamination by radioactive particles and gases.

There should be a system to prevent air entering the clean area through extract ducts e.g. when the extract fan is not operating.

Production

6. Production of different radioactive products in the same work stations and at the same time should be avoided in order to minimize the risk of cross-contamination or mix-up.

7. Process validation, in-process controls and monitoring of process parameters and environment assume particular importance in cases where it is necessary to take the decision to release or reject a batch or a product before all tests are completed.

Quality control

8. When products have to be dispatched before all tests are completed, this does not obviate the need for a formal recorded decision to be taken by the Qualified Person on the conformity of the batch. In this case there should be a written procedure detailing all production and Quality Control data which should be considered before the batch is dispatched. A procedure should also describe the measures to be taken by the Qualified Person if unsatisfactory test results are obtained after dispatch.

9. Unless otherwise specified in the marketing authorization, reference samples of every batch should be retained.

Distribution and recalls

10. Detailed distribution records should be maintained and there should be procedures which describe the measures to be taken in for stopping the use of defective radiopharmaceuticals. Recall operations should be shown to be operable within a very short time.

ANNEX 4 MANUFACTURE OF VETERINARY MEDICINAL PRODUCTS OTHER THAN IMMUNOLOGICAL VETERINARY MEDICINAL PRODUCTS

Note

This annex applies to all veterinary medicinal products falling within the scope of Directive 81/851/EEC other than immunological veterinary medicinal products, which are the subject of a separate annex.

Manufacture of premixes for medicated feedingstuffs

For the purposes of these paragraphs,

- *a medicated feedingstuff* is any mixture of a veterinary medicinal product or products and feed or feeds which is ready prepared for marketing and intended to be fed to animals without further processing because of its curative or preventative properties or other properties as a medicinal product covered by Article 1(2) of Directive 65/65/EEC;

- *a pre-mix for medicated feedingstuffs* is any veterinary medicinal product prepared in advance with a view to the subsequent manufacture of medicated feedingstuffs.

1. The manufacture of premixes for medicated feedingstuffs requires the use of large quantities of vegetable matter which is likely to attract insects and rodents. Premises should be designed, equipped and operated to minimize this risk (point 3.4.) and should also be subject to a regular pest control programme.

2. Because of the large volume of dust generated during the production of bulk material for premixes, specific attention should be given to the need to avoid cross contamination and facilitate cleaning (point 3.14), for example through the installation of sealed transport systems and dust extraction, whenever possible. The installation of such systems does not, however, eliminate the need for regular cleaning of production areas.

3. Parts of the process likely to have a significant adverse influence on the stability of the active ingredient(s) (e.g. use of steam in pellet manufacture) should be carried out in a uniform manner from batch to batch.

4. Consideration should be given to undertake the manufacture of premixes in dedicated areas which, if at all possible, do not form part of a main manufacturing plant. Alternatively, such dedicated areas should be surrounded by a buffer zone in order to minimize the risk of contamination of other manufacturing areas.

The manufacture of ectoparasiticides

5. In derogation from point 3.6, ectoparasiticides for external application to animals, which are veterinary medicinal products, and subject to marketing authorization, may be produced and filled on a compaign basis in pesticide specific areas. However other categories of veterinary medicinal products should not be produced in such areas.

6. Adequate validated cleaning procedures should be employed to prevent cross contamination, and steps should be taken to ensure the secure storage of the veterinary medicinal product in accordance with the guide.

The manufacture of veterinary medicinal products containing penicillins

7. The use of penicillins in veterinary medicine does not present the same risks of hypersensitivity in animals as in humans. Although incidents of hypersensitivity have been recorded in horses and dogs, there are other materials which are toxic to certain species, e.g. the ionophore antibiotics in horses. Although desirable, the requirements that such products be manufactured in dedicated, self-contained facilities (point 3.6) may be dispensed with in the case of facilities dedicated to the manufacture of veterinary medicinal products only. However, all necessary measures should be taken to avoid cross contamination and any risk to operator safety in accordance with the guide. In such circumstances, penicillin-containing products should be manufactured on a campaign basis and should be followed by appropriate, validated decontamination and cleaning procedures.

Retention of samples (point 1.4. viii and point 6.14.)

8. It is recognized that because of the large volume of certain veterinary medicinal products in their final packaging, in particular premixes, it may not be feasible for manufacturers to retain samples from each batch in its final packaging. However, manufacturers should ensure that sufficient representative samples of each batch are retained and stored in accordance with the guide.

9. In all cases, the container used for storage should be composed of the same material as the market primary container in which the product is marketed.

Sterile veterinary medicinal products

10. Where this has been accepted by the competent authorities, terminally sterilized veterinary medicinal products may be manufactured in a clean area of a lower grade than the grade required in the annex on "Sterile preparations", but at least in a grade D environment.

ANNEX 5 MANUFACTURE OF IMMUNOLOGICAL VETERINARY MEDICINAL PRODUCTS

Principle

The manufacture of immunological veterinary medicinal products has special characteristics which should be taken into consideration when implementing and assessing the quality assurance system.

Due to the large number of animal species and related pathogenic agents, the variety of products manufactured is very wide and the volume of manufacture is often low; hence, work on a compaign basis is common. Moreover, because of the very nature of this manufacture (cultivation steps, lack of terminal sterilization, etc), the products must be particularly well-protected against contamination and cross-contamination. The environment also must be protected especially when the manufacture involves the use of pathogenic or exotic biological agents and the worker must be particularly well-protected when the manufacture involves the use of biological agents pathogenic to man.

These factors, together with the inherent variability of immunological products and the relative inefficiency in particular of final product quality control tests in providing adequate information about products, means that the role of the quality assurance system is of the utmost importance. The need to maintain control over all of the following aspects of GMP, as well as those outlined in this Guide, cannot be overemphasized. In particular, it is important that the data generated by the monitoring of the various aspects of GMP (equipment, premises, product etc.) are rigorously assessed and informed decisions, leading to appropriate action, are made and recorded.

Personnel

1. All personnel (including those concerned with cleaning and maintenance) employed in areas where immunological products are manufactured should be given training in and information on hygiene and microbiology. They should receive additional training specific to the products with which they work.

2. Responsible personnel should be formally trained in some or all of the following fields: bacteriology, biology, biometry, chemistry, immunology, medicine, parasitology, pharmacy, pharmacology, virology and veterinary medicine and should also have an adequate knowledge of environmental protection measures.

3. Personnel should be protected against possible infection with the biological agents used in manufacture. In the case of biological agents known to cause disease in humans, adequate measures should be taken to prevent infection of personnel working with the agent or with experimental animals.

Where relevant, the personnel should be vaccinated and subject to medical examination.

4. Adequate measures should be taken to prevent biological agents being taken outside the manufacturing plant by personnel acting as a carrier. Dependent on the type of biological agent, such measures may include complete change of clothes and compulsory showering before leaving the production area.

5. For immunological products, the risk of contamination or cross-contamination by personnel is particularly important.

   Prevention of *contamination* by personnel should be achieved by a set of measures and procedures to ensure that appropriate protective clothing is used during the different stages of the production process.

   Prevention of *cross-contamination* by personnel involved in production should be achieved by a set of measures and procedures to ensure that they do not pass from one area to another unless they have taken appropriate measures to eliminate the risk of contamination. In the course of a working day, personnel should not pass from areas where contamination with live microorganisms is likely or where animals are housed to premises where other products or organisms are handled. If such passage is unavoidable, clearly defined decontamination procedures, including change of clothing and shoes, and, where necessary, showering, should be followed by staff involved in any such production.

   Personnel entering a contained area where organisms had not been handled in open circuit operations in the previous twelve hours to check on cultures in sealed, surface decontaminated flasks would not be regarded as being at risk of contamination, unless the organism involved was an exotic.

Premises

6. Premises should be designed in such a way as to control both the risk to the product and to the environment.

   This can be achieved by the use of containment, clean, clean/contained or controlled areas.

7. Live biological agents should be handled in contained areas. The level of containment should depend on the pathogenicity of the microorganism and whether it has been classified as exotic. (Other relevant legislation, such as Directives 90/219/EEC and 90/220/EEC, also applies).

8. Inactivated biological agents should be handled in clean areas. Clean areas should also be used when handling non-infected cells isolated from multicellular organisms and, in some cases, filtration-sterilized media.

9. Open circuit operations involving products or components not subsequently sterilised should be carried out within a laminar air flow work station (grade A) in a grade B area.

10. Other operations where live biological agents are handled (quality control, research and diagnostic services, etc) should be appropriately contained and separated if production operations are carried out in the same building. The level of containment should depend on the pathogenicity of the biological agent and whether they have been classified as exotic. Whenever diagnostic activities are carried out, there is the risk of introducing highly pathogenic organisms. Therefore, the level of containment should be adequate to cope with all such risks. Containment may also be required if quality control or other activities are carried out in buildings in close proximity to those used for production.

11. Containment premises should be easily disinfected and should have the following characteristics:
    (a) The absence of direct venting to the outside;
    (b) a ventilation with air at negative pressure. Air should be extracted through HEPA filters and not be recirculated except to the same area, and provided further HEPA filtration is used (normally this condition would be met by routing the recirculated air through the normal supply HEPAs for that area). However, recycling of air between areas may be permissible provided that it passes through two exhaust HEPAs, the first of which is continuously monitored for integrity, and there are adequate measures for safe venting of exhaust air should this filter fail;
    (c) air from manufacturing areas used for the handling of exotic organisms should be vented through 2 sets of HEPA filters in series, and that from production areas not recirculated;
    (d) a system for the collection and disinfection of liquid effluents including contaminated condensate from sterilizers, biogenerators, etc. Solid wastes, including animal carcasses, should be disinfected, sterilized or incinerated as appropriate. Contaminated filters should be removed using a safe method;
    (e) changing rooms designed and used as air locks, and equipped with washing and showering facilities if appropriate. Air pressure differentials should be such that there is no flow of air between the work area and the external environment or risk of contamination of outer clothing worn outside the area;
    (f) an air lock system for the passage of equipment, which is constructed so that there is no flow of contaminated air between the work area and the external environment or risk of contamination of equipment within the lock. The air lock should be of a size which enables the effective surface decontamination of materials being passed through it. Consideration should be given to having a timing device on the door interlock to allow sufficient time for the decontamination process to be effective.
    (g) in many instances, a barrier double-door autoclave for the secure removal of waste materials and introduction of sterile items.

12. Equipment passes and changing rooms should have an interlock mechanism or other appropriate system to prevent the opening of more than one door at a time. Changing rooms should be supplied with air filtered to the same standard as that for the work area, and equipped with air extraction facilities to produce an adequate air circulation independent of that of the work area. Equipment passes should normally be ventilated in the same way, but unventilated passes, or those equipped with supply air only, may be acceptable.

13. Production operations such as cell maintenance, media preparation, virus culture, etc. likely to cause contamination should be performed in separate areas. Animals and animal products should be handled with appropriate precautions.

14. Production areas where biological agents particularly resistant to disinfection (e.g. spore-forming bacteria) are handled should be separated and dedicated to that particular purpose until the biological agents have been inactivated.

15. With the exception of blending and subsequent filling operations, one biological agent only should be handled at a time within an area.

16. Production areas should be designed to permit disinfection between campaigns, using validated methods.

17. Production of biological agents may take place in controlled areas provided it is carried out in totally enclosed and heat sterilized equipment, all connections being also heat sterilized after making and before breaking. It may be acceptable for connections to be made under local laminar air flow provided these are few in number and proper aseptic techniques are used and there is no risk of leakage. The sterilization parameters used before breaking the connections must be validated for the organisms being used. Different products may be placed in different biogenerators, within the same area, provided that there is no risk of accidental cross-contamination. However, organisms generally subject to special requirements for containment should be in areas dedicated to such products.

18. Animal houses where animals intended or used for production are accommodated, should be provided with the appropriate containment and/or clean area measures, and should be separate from other animal accommodation.

Animal houses where animals used for quality control, involving the use of pathogenic biological agents, are accommodated, should be adequately contained.

19. Access to manufacturing areas should be restricted to authorized personnel. Clear and concise written procedures should be posted as appropriate.

20. Documentation relating to the premises should be readily available in a plant master file.

The manufacturing site and buildings should be described in sufficient detail (by means of plans and written explanations) so that the designation and conditions of use of all the rooms are correctly identified as well as the biological agents which are handled in them. The flow of people and product should also be clearly marked.

The animal species accommodated in the animal houses or otherwise on the site should be identified.

The activities carried out in the vicinity of the site should also be indicated.

Plans of contained and/or clean area premises, should describe the ventilation system indicating inlets and outlets, filters and their specifications, the number of air changes per hour, and pressure gradients. They should indicate which pressure gradients are monitored by pressure indicator.

Equipment

21. The equipment used should be designed and constructed so that it meets the particular requirements for the manufacture of each product.

    Before being put into operation the equipment should be qualified and validated and subsequently be regularly maintained and validated.

22. Where appropriate, the equipment should ensure satisfactory primary containment of the biological agents.

    Where appropriate, the equipment should be designed and constructed as to allow easy and effective decontamination and/or sterilization.

23. Closed equipment used for the primary containment of the biological agents should be designed and constructed as to prevent any leakage or the formation of droplets and aerosols.

    Inlets and outlets for gases should be protected so as to achieve adequate containment e.g. by the use of sterilizing hydrophobic filters.

    The introduction or removal of material should take place using a sterilizable closed system, or possibly in an appropriate laminar air flow.

24. Equipment where necessary should be properly sterilized before use, preferably by pressurized dry steam. Other methods can be accepted if steam sterilization cannot be used because of the nature of the equipment. It is important not to overlook such individual items as bench centrifuges and water baths.

    Equipment used for purification, separation or concentration should be sterilized or disinfected at least between use for different products. The effect of the sterilization methods on the effectiveness and validity of the equipment should be studied in order to determine the life span of the equipment.

    All sterilization procedures should be validated

25. Equipment should be designed so as to prevent any mix-up between different organisms or products. Pipes, valves and filters should be identified as to their function.

Separate incubators should be used for infected and non infected containers and also generally for different organisms or cells. Incubators containing more than one organism or cell type will only be acceptable if adequate steps are taken to seal, surface decontaminate and segregate the containers. Culture vessels, etc. should be individually labelled. The cleaning and disinfection of the items can be particularly difficult and should receive special attention.

Equipment used for the storage of biological agents or products should be designed and used in such a manner as to prevent any possible mix-up. All stored items should be clearly and unambiguously labelled and in leak-proof containers. Items such as cells and organisms seed stock should be stored in dedicated equipment.

26. Relevant equipment, such as that requiring temperature control, should be fitted with recording and/or alarm systems.

To avoid breakdowns, a system of preventive maintenance, together with trend analysis of recorded data, should be implemented.

27. The loading of freeze driers requires an appropriate clean/contained area.

Unloading freeze driers contaminates the immediate environment. Therefore, for single-ended freeze driers, the clean room should be decontaminated before a further manufacturing batch is introduced into the area, unless this contains the same organisms, and double door freeze driers should be sterilized after each cycle unless opened in a clean area.

Sterilization of freeze driers should be done in accordance with item 24. In case of campaign working, they should at least be sterilized after each campaign.

Animals and animal houses

28. General requirements for animal quarters, care and quarantine are laid down in Directive 86/609/EEC.

29. Animal houses should be separated from the other production premises and suitably designed.

30. The sanitary status of the animals used for production should be defined, monitored, and recorded. Some animals should be handled as defined in specific monographs (e.g. Specific Pathogens Free flocks).

31. Animals, biological agents, and tests carried out should be the subject of an identification system so as to prevent any risk of confusion and to control all possible hazards.

Disinfection – Waste disposal

32. Disinfection and/or wastes and effluents disposal may be particularly important in the case of manufacture of immunological products. Careful consideration should therefore be given to procedures and equipment aiming at avoiding environmental contamination as well as to their validation or qualification.

Production

33. Because of the wide variety of products, the frequently large number of stages involved in the manufacture of immunological veterinary medicinal products and the nature of the biological processes, careful attention must be paid to adherence to validated operating procedures, to the constant monitoring of production at all stages and to in-process controls.

    Additionally, special consideration should be given to starting materials, media and the use of a seed lot system.

Starting materials

34. The suitability of starting materials should be clearly defined in written specifications. These should include details of the supplier, the method of manufacture, the geographical origin and the animal species from which the materials are derived. The controls to be applied to starting materials must be included. Microbiological controls are particulary important.

35. The results of tests on starting materials must comply with the specifications. Where the tests take a long time (e.g. eggs from SPF flocks) it may be necessary to process starting materials before the results of analytical controls are available. In such cases, the release of a finished product is conditional upon satisfactory results of the tests on starting materials.

36. Special attention should be paid to a knowledge of the supplier's quality assurance system in assessing the suitability of a source and the extent of quality control testing required.

37. Where possible, heat is the preferred method for sterilizing starting materials. If necessary, other validated methods, such as irradiation, may be used.

Media

38. The ability of media to support the desired growth should be properly validated in advance.

39. Media should preferably be sterilized in situ or in line. Heat is the preferred method. Gases, media, acids, alkalis, defoaming agents and other materials introduced into sterile biogenerators should themselves be sterile.

Seed lot and cell bank system

40. In order to prevent the unwanted drift of properties which might ensue from repeated subcultures or multiple generations, the production of immunological veterinary medicinal products obtained by microbial, cell or tissue culture, or propagation in embryos and animals, should be based on a system of seed lots or cell banks.

41. The number of generations (doublings, passages) between the seed lot or cell bank and the finished product should be consistent with the dossier of authorization for marketing.

42. Seed lots and cell banks should be adequately characterized and tested for contaminants. Acceptance criteria for new seed lots should be established. Seed lots and cell banks shall be established, stored and used in such a way as to minimize the risks of contamination, or any alteration. During the establishment of the seed lot and cell bank, no other living or infectious material (e.g. virus or cell lines) shall be handled simultaneously in the same area or by the same person.

43. Establishment of the seed lot and cell bank should be performed in a suitable environment to protect the seed lot and the cell bank and, if applicable, the personnel handling it and the external environment.

44. The origin, form and storage conditions of seed material should be described in full. Evidence of the stability and recovery of the seeds and cells should be provided. Storage containers should be hermetically sealed, clearly labelled and stored at an appropriate temperature. Storage conditions shall be properly monitored. An inventory should be kept and each container accounted for.

45. Only authorized personnel should be allowed to handle the material and this handling should be done under the supervision of a responsible person. Different seed lots or cell banks shall be stored in such a way to avoid confusion or cross-contamination errors. It is desirable to split the seed lots and cell banks and to store the parts at different locations so as to minimize the risk of total loss.

Operating principles

46. The formation of droplets and the production of foam should be avoided or minimized during manufacturing processes. Centrifugation and blending procedures which can lead to droplet formation should be carried out in appropriate contained or clean/contained areas to prevent transfer of live organisms.

47. Accidental spillages, especially of live organisms, must be dealt with quickly and safely. Validated decontamination measures should be available for each organism.

Where different strains of single bacteria species or very similar viruses are involved, the process need be validated against only one of them, unless there is reason to believe that they may vary significantly in their resistance to the agent(s) involved.

48. Operations involving the transfer of materials such as sterile media, cultures or product should be carried out in pre-sterilized closed systems wherever possible. Where this is not possible, transfer operations must be protected by laminar airflow work stations.

49. Addition of media or cultures to biogenerators and other vessels should be carried out under carefully controlled conditions to ensure that contamination is not introduced. Care must be taken to ensure that vessels are correctly connected when addition of cultures takes place.

50. Where necessary, for instance when two or more fermentors are within a single area, sampling and addition ports, and connectors (after connection, before the flow of product, and again before disconnection) should be sterilized with steam. In other circumstances, chemical disinfection of ports and laminar air flow protection of connections may be acceptable.

51. Equipment, glassware, the external surfaces of product containers and other such materials must be disinfected before transfer from a contained area using a validated method (see 47 above). Batch documentation can be a particular problem. Only the absolute minimum required to a low operations to GMP standards should enter and leave the area. If obviously contaminated, such as by spills or aerosols, or if the organism involved is an exotic, the paperwork must be adequately disinfected through an equipment pass, or the information transferred out by such means as photocopy or fax.

52. Liquid or solid wastes such as the debris after harvesting eggs, disposable culture bottles, unwanted cultures or biological agents, are best sterilized or disinfected before transfer from a contained area. However, alternatives such as sealed containers or piping may be appropriate in some cases.

53. Articles and materials, including documentation, entering a production room should be carefully controlled to ensure that only articles and materials concerned with production are introduced. There should be a system which ensures that articles and materials entering a room are reconciled with those leaving so that their accumulation within the room does not occur.

54. Heat stable articles and materials entering a clean area or clean/contained area should do so through a double-ended autoclave or oven. Heat labile articles and materials should enter through an air-lock with interlocked doors where they are disinfected. Sterilization of articles and materials elsewhere is acceptable provided that they are double wrapped and enter through an airlock with the appropriate precautions.

55. Precautions must be taken to avoid contamination or confusion during incubation. There should be a cleaning and disinfection procedure for incubators. Containers in incubators should be carefully and clearly labelled.

56. With the exception of blending and subsequent filling operations (or when totally enclosed systems are used) only one live biological agent may be handled within a production room at any given time. Production rooms must be effectively disinfected between the handling of different live biological agents.

57. Products should be inactivated by the addition of inactivant accompanied by sufficient agitation. The mixture should then be transferred to a second sterile vessel, unless the container is of such a size and shape as to be easily inverted and shaken so as to wet all internal surfaces with the final culture/inactivant mixture.

58. Vessels containing inactivated product should not be opened or sampled in areas containing live biological agents. All subsequent processing of inactivated products should take place in clean areas grade A–B or enclosed equipment dedicated to inactivated products.

59. Careful consideration should be given to the validation of methods for sterilization, disinfection, virus removal and inactivation.

60. Filling should be carried out as soon as possible following production. Containers of bulk product prior to filling should be sealed, appropriately labelled and stored under specified conditions of temperature.

61. There should be a system to assure the integrity and closure of containers after filling.

62. The capping of vials containing live biological agents must be performed in such a way that ensures that contamination of other products or escape of the live agents into other areas or the external environment does not occur.

63. For various reasons there may be a delay between the filling of final containers and their labelling and packaging. Procedures should be specified for the storage of unlabelled containers in order to prevent confusion and to ensure satisfactory storage conditions. Special attention should be paid to the storage of heat labile or photosensitive products. Storage temperatures should be specified.

64. For each stage of production, the yield of product should be reconciled with that expected from that process. Any significant discrepancies should be investigated.

Quality control

65. In-process controls play a specially important role in ensuring the consistency of the quality of biological medicinal products. Those controls which are crucial for the

quality (e.g. virus removal) but which cannot be carried out on the finished product, should be performed at an appropriate stage of production.

66. It may be necessary to retain samples of intermediate products in sufficient amount and under appropriate storage conditions to allow repetition or confirmation of a batch control.

67. There may be a requirement for the continuous monitoring of data during a production process, for example monitoring of physical parameters during fermentation.

68. Continuous culture of biological products is a common practice and special consideration needs to be given to the quality control requirements arising from this type of production method.

ANNEX 6 MANUFACTURE OF MEDICINAL GASES

Because the manufacture of medicinal gases is a specialized industrial process not normally undertaken by pharmaceutical companies, manufacturers of these gases are not always familiar with the regulatory provisions governing the pharmaceutical industry. Medicinal gases are nevertheless classified as medicinal products, and their manufacture should comply with good manufacturing practice.

Personnel

1. The qualified person responsible for releasing batches should have a thorough knowledge of the production and control of medicinal gases including practical experience. All personnel should know the GMP relevant to medicinal gases and should be aware of the critically important aspects and potential hazards for patients from medicinal products in the form of gas.

Premises and equipment

2. The manufacture of medicinal gases is generally carried out in closed equipment. Consequently, environmental contamination of the product is minimal. However, there is a risk of cross-contamination with other gases.

3. Premises should provide sufficient space for manufacturing, filling and testing operations to avoid the risk of mix-up. Premises should be clean and tidy to encourage orderly working.

4. Filling areas should be of sufficient size and have an orderly layout to provide:
   (a) separate marked areas for different gases and different cylinder sizes;
   (b) clearly identifiable segregation of empty cylinders from full cylinders;
   (c) clear distinction of the stage reached by given cylinders (e.g. "awaiting filling", "filled", "awaiting test", "released").

   The method used to achieve these various levels of segregation will depend on the nature, extent and complexity of the overall operation, but marked-out floor areas, partitions, barriers, labels and signs should be used as appropriate.

5. It is necessary to ensure that the correct gas is put into the correct container. There should be no interconnections between pipelines carrying different gases. The manifolds should be equipped with fill connections that correspond only to the valve for that particular gas or mixture of gases so that the wrong containers cannot be attached to the manifold. (The use of manifold and container valve connections may be subject to national or international rules.)

6. Repair and maintenance operations should not present any hazard to the quality of the medicinal gas.

7. Medicinal gases should be filled in a separate area from non medicinal gases and there should be no exchange of cylinders between these areas.

8. It may be acceptable to fill non medicinal and medicinal gases cylinders (concurrently) on the same line but in different areas, provided that the gas used for non medicinal purposes is at least equal to the quality of the medicinal gas, and the cylinders have been prepared in accordance with specific requirements referred to in this supplementary guide. There should be a non return valve in the line supplying the filling area for non medicinal gases to prevent contamination.

9. Cylinders for medicinal gases should have appropriate technical characteristics. The outlets of cylinders should be equipped with tamper-evident seals.

10. Liquefied refrigerated medicinal gas may be transported in the same tankers as the same non medicinal gas provided that the latter is at least equal quality to the medicinal gas.

Production and Quality Control

11. Gas production should be continuously monitored for quality and impurity levels.

12. All the transfer operations of liquefied refrigerated medicinal gases from primary storage should be in accordance with a written procedure designed to avoid any contamination.

13. Deliveries of gas may be added to bulk storage tanks containing the same gas from previous deliveries. In this case, either:
    - a sample must be tested and found acceptable before the delivery is added; or
    - when the finished product is a single gas the sample may be taken either from the mixed delivery in the bulk storage tank or from the first cylinder filled, provided that the filling line has been purged after the new shipment has been added to the bulk tank;
    - when the finished product is a mixture of gases, each component should be tested separately.

14. The medicinal gases manifold should be dedicated to a single gas or to a given mixture of gases.

15. Cleaning and purging of filling equipment and pipelines should follow written procedures, and checks for the absence of cleaning agents or other contaminants should be carried out before the line is released for use.

16. New cylinders and cylinders returned to use after any pressure test should be subject to an internal visual inspection.

17. Checks to be performed before filling should include:
   - visual external inspection of each valve and container for dents, arc burns, other damage and oil or grease;
   - a check of each cylinder or cryogenic vessel valve connection to determine that it is the proper type for the particular medicinal gas involved;
   - a check to determine that the hydrostatic test has been conducted as required. Each cylinder should be coded to show the date of the last hydrostatic test;
   - a check to determine that each container is colour-coded and labelled.

18. Cylinders which have been returned for refilling should be prepared as follows: any gas remaining in the cylinders should be removed by blowing down each container, followed by a purge (partial pressurisation then blowing down) or evacuation of the container [at least 25 inches of mercury – i.e. absolute pressure below 150 mbar]. As an alternative, full analysis of the remaining gas should be carried out for each individual container. Consideration should also be given to inversion of the container while blowing down to assist with the removal of any liquid contaminant.

19. There should be appropriate checks to ensure that containers have been filled.

20. In the case of a single medicinal gas filled via a multi-cylinder manifold, at least one cylinder of product from each manifold filling should be tested for identity and purity each time the cylinders are changed on the manifold.

21. In the case of a single medicinal gas put into cylinders one at a time by individual filling operations, at least one cylinder of each uninterrupted filling cycle should be tested for identity and assay. An example of an uninterrupted filling operation cycle is one shift's production using the same personnel, equipment, and batch of bulk gas.

22. In the case of a finished product gas produced by mixing two different gases in a cylinder, every cylinder should be tested for the identity and assay of one of the gases, and at least one cylinder from each manifold filling should be tested for identity of the other gas in the mixture.

23. In the case of a finished medicinal gas produced by mixing three different gases in a cylinder, every cylinder should be tested for the identity and assay of two of the gases and at least one cylinder from each manifold filling should be tested for the identity of the third gas in the mixture.

    When gases are mixed in-line before filling (e.g. nitrous oxide/oxygen mixture) continuous analysis of the mixture being filled is required.

24. When a cylinder is filled with more than one gas, the filling process must ensure that the gases are correctly mixed in every cylinder and are fully homogeneous.

25. Each filled cylinder should be tested for leaks using an appropriate method, such as a leak detection solution applied to the valve area.

26. In the case of cryogenic liquefied gas filled into cryogenic vessels for delivery to users, each vessel should be tested for identity and assay.

27. Cryogenic vessels which are retained by customers and refilled in place from mobile delivery tanks need not be sampled after filling provided the filling company delivers a certificate of analysis for a sample taken from their tank.

28. Retained samples are not required, unless otherwise specified.

Labelling

29. Each cylinder should be labelled and colour-coded. The batch number may be on a separate label.

Storage – Release

30. Following filling, all cylinders should be held in quarantine until released by the qualified person.

31. Gas cylinders should be stored under cover and not be subjected to extremes of temperature. Storage areas should be clean, dry, well ventilated and free of combustible materials.

32. Storage arrangements should permit segregation of different gases and of full/empty cylinders and permit rotation of stock.

ANNEX 7 MANUFACTURE OF HERBAL MEDICINAL PRODUCTS

Principle

Because of their often complex and variable nature, and the number and small quantity of defined active ingredients, control of starting materials, storage and processing assume particular importance in the manufacture of herbal medicinal products.

Premises

Storage areas

1. Crude (i.e. unprocessed) plants should be stored in separate areas. The storage area should be well ventilated and be equipped in such a way as to give protection against the entry of insects or other animals, especially rodents. Effective measures should be taken to prevent the spread of any such animals and microorganisms brought in with the crude plant and to prevent cross-contamination. Containers should be located in such a way as to allow free air circulation.

2. Special attention should be paid to the cleanliness and good maintenance of the storage areas particularly when dust is generated.

3. Storage of plants, extracts, tinctures and other preparations may require special conditions of humidity, temperature or light protection; these conditions should be provided and monitored.

Production area

4. Specific provisions should be taken during sampling, weighing, mixing and processing operations of crude plants whenever dust is generated, to facilitate cleaning and to avoid cross-contamination, as for example, dust extraction, dedicated premises, etc.

Documentation

Specifications for starting materials

5. Apart from the data described in General Guide (chapter 4, point 4.11), specifications for medicinal crude plants should include, as far as possible:
   - the botanical name (with, if appropriate, the name of the originator of the classification, e.g. Linnaeus);
   - the details of the source of the plant (country or region of origin, and where applicable, cultivation, time of harvesting, collection procedures, possible pesticides used, etc.);

- whether the whole plant or only a part is used;
- when a dried plant is purchased, the drying system should be specified;
- the description of the plant and its macro and microscopical examination;
- the suitable identification tests including, where appropriate, identification tests for known active ingredients, or markers. A reference authentic specimen should be available for identification purposes;
- the assay, where appropriate, of constituents of known therapeutic activity or of markers;
- the methods suitable to determine possible pesticide contamination and limits accepted;
- the tests to determine fungal and/or microbial contamination, including aflatoxins and pest-infestations, and limits accepted;
- the tests for toxic metals and for likely contaminants and adulterants;
- the tests for foreign materials.

Any treatment used to reduce fungal/microbial contamination or other infestation should be documented. Specifications for such procedures should be available and should include details of process, tests and limits for residues.

Processing instructions

6. The processing instructions should describe the different operations carried out upon the crude plant such as drying, crushing and sifting, and include drying time and temperatures, and methods used to control fragment or particle size. It should also describe security sieving or other methods of removing foreign materials.

   For the production of a vegetable drug preparation, instructions should include details of base or solvent, time and temperatures of extraction, details of any concentration stages and methods used (see also the note for guidance "Quality of herbal remedies", Volume III of "The rules governing medicinal products in the European Community").

Sampling

7. Due to the fact that crude drugs are an aggregate of individual plants and contain an element of heterogeneity, their sampling has to be carried out with special care by personnel with particular expertise. Each batch should be identified by its own documentation.

Quality Control

8. Quality Control personnel should have particular expertise in herbal medicinal products in order to be able to carry out identification tests and recognize adulteration,

the presence of fungal growth, infestations, non-uniformity within a delivery of crude plants, etc.

9. The identity and quality of vegetable drug preparations and of finished product should be tested as described in the note for guidance "Quality of herbal remedies".

ANNEX 8 SAMPLING OF STARTING AND PACKAGING MATERIALS

Principle

Sampling is an important operation in which only a small fraction of a batch is taken. Valid conclusions on the whole cannot be based on tests which have been carried out on non-representative samples. Correct sampling is thus an essential part of a system of Quality Assurance.

Note

Sampling is dealt with in Chapter 6 of the Guide, items 6.11. to 6.14. This annex gives additional guidance on the sampling of starting and packaging materials.

Personnel

1. Personnel who take samples should receive initial and on-going regular training in the disciplines relevant to correct sampling. This training should include:
   - sampling plans,
   - written sampling procedures,
   - the techniques and equipment for sampling,
   - the risks of cross-contamination,
   - the precautions to be taken with regard to unstable and/or sterile substances,
   - the importance of considering the visual appearance of materials, containers and labels,
   - the importance of recording any unexpected or unusual circumstances.

Starting materials

2. The identity of a complete batch of starting materials can normally only be ensured if individual samples are taken from all the containers and an identity test performed on each sample. It is permissible to sample only a proportion of the containers where a validated procedure has been established to ensure that no single container of starting material has been incorrectly labelled.

3. This validation should take account of at least the following aspects:
   - the nature and status of the manufacturer and of the supplier and their understanding of the GMP requirements of the Pharmaceutical Industry;
   - the Quality Assurance system of the manufacturer of the starting material;
   - the manufacturing conditions under which the starting material is produced and controlled;

- the nature of the starting material and the medicinal products in which it will be used.

Under such a system, it is possible that a validated procedure exempting identity testing of each incoming container of starting material could be accepted for:

- starting materials coming from a single product manufacturer or plant;
- starting materials coming directly from a manufacturer or in the manufacturer's sealed container where there is a history of reliability and regular audits of the manufacturer's Quality Assurance system are conducted by the purchaser (the manufacturer of the medicinal product) or by an officially accredited body.

It is improbable that a procedure could be satisfactorily validated for:

- starting materials supplied by intermediaries such as brokers where the source of manufacture is unknown or not audited;
- starting materials for use in parenteral products.

4. The quality of a batch of starting materials may be assessed by taking and testing a representative sample. The samples taken for identity testing could be used for this purpose. The number of samples taken for the preparation of a representative sample should be determined statistically and specified in a sampling plan. The number of individual samples which may be blended to form a composite sample should also be defined, taking into account the nature of the material, knowledge of the supplier and the homogeneity of the composite sample.

Packaging Material

5. The sampling plan for packaging materials should take account of at least the following: the quantity received, the quality required, the nature of the material (e.g. primary packaging materials and/or printed packaging materials), the production methods, and what is known of the Quality Assurance system of the packaging materials manufacturer based on audits. The number of samples taken should be determined statistically and specified in a sampling plan.

ANNEX 9 MANUFACTURE OF LIQUIDS, CREAMS AND OINTMENTS

Principle

Liquids, creams and ointments may be particularly susceptible to microbial and other contamination during manufacture. Therefore special measures must be taken to prevent any contamination.

Premises and Equipment

1. The use of closed systems for processing and transfer is recommended in order to protect the product from contamination. Production areas where the products or open clean containers are exposed should normally be effectively ventilated with filtered air.

2. Tanks, containers, pipework and pumps should be designed and installed so that they may be readily cleaned and if necessary sanitized. In particular, equipment design should include a minimum of dead-legs or sites where residues can accumulate and promote microbial proliferation.

3. The use of glass apparatus should be avoided wherever possible. High quality stainless steel is often the material of choice for parts coming into contact with product.

Production

4. The chemical and microbiological quality of water used in production should be specified and monitored. Care should be taken in the maintenance of water systems in order to avoid the risk of microbial proliferation. After any chemical sanitization of the water systems, a validated flushing procedure should be followed to ensure that the sanitizing agent has been effectively removed.

5. The quality of materials received in bulk tankers should be checked before they are transferred to bulk storage tanks.

6. Care should be taken when transferring materials via pipelines to ensure that they are delivered to their correct destination.

7. Materials likely to shed fibres or other contaminants, like cardboard or wooden pallets, should not enter the areas where products or clean containers are exposed.

8. Care should be taken to maintain the homogeneity of mixtures, suspensions, etc. during filling. Mixing and filling processes should be validated. Special care should be taken at the beginning of a filling process, after stoppages and at the end of the process to ensure that homogeneity is maintained.

9. When the finished product is not immediately packaged, the maximum period of storage and the storage conditions should be specified and adhered to.

ANNEX 10 MANUFACTURE OF PRESSURIZED METERED DOSE AEROSOL PREPARATIONS FOR INHALATION

Principle

The manufacture of pressurized aerosol products for inhalation with metering valves requires special consideration because of the particular nature of this form of product. It should be done under conditions which minimize microbial and particulate contamination. Assurance of the quality of the valve components and, in the case of suspensions, of uniformity is also of particular importance.

General

1. There are presently two common manufacturing and filling methods as follows:
   a. Two-shot system (pressure filling). The active ingredient is suspended in a high boiling point propellant, the dose is put into the container, the valve is crimped on and the lower boiling point propellant is injected through the valve stem to make up the finished product. The suspension of active ingredient in propellant is kept cool to reduce evaporation loss.
   b. One-shot process (cold filling). The active ingredient is suspended in a mixture of propellants and held either under high pressure or at a low temperature, or both. The suspension is then filled directly into the container in one shot.

Premises and Equipment

2. Manufacture and filling should be carried out as far as possible in a closed system.

3. Where products or clean components are exposed, the area should be fed with filtered air, should comply with the requirements of at least a Grade D environment and should be entered through airlocks.

Production and Quality Control

4. Metering valves for aerosols are more complex pieces of engineering than most items used in pharmaceutical production. Their specifications, sampling and testing should recognize this. Auditing the Quality Assurance system of the valve manufacturer is of particular importance.

5. All fluids (e.g. liquid or gaseous propellants) should be filtered to remove particles greater than 0.2 micron. An additional filtration where possible immediately before filling is desirable.

6. Containers and valves should be cleaned using a validated procedure appropriate to the use of the product to ensure the absence of any contaminants such as fabrication aids (e.g. lubricants) or undue microbiological contaminants. After cleaning, valves should be kept in clean, closed containers and precautions taken not to introduce contamination during subsequent handling, e.g. taking samples. Containers should be fed to the filling line in a clean condition or cleaned on line immediately before filling.

7. Precautions should be taken to ensure uniformity of suspensions at the point of fill throughout the filling process.

8. When a two-shot filling process is used, it is necessary to ensure that both shots are of the correct weight in order to achieve the correct composition. For this purpose, 100% weight checking at each stage is often desirable.

9. Controls after filling should ensure the absence of undue leakage. Any leakage test should be performed in a way which avoids microbial contamination or residual moisture.

ANNEX 11 COMPUTERIZED SYSTEMS

Principle

The introduction of computerized systems into systems of manufacturing, including storage, distribution and quality control does not alter the need to observe the relevant principles given elsewhere in the Guide. Where a computerized system replaces a manual operation, there should be no resultant decrease in product quality or quality assurance. Consideration should be given to the risk of losing aspects of the previous system which could result from reducing the involvement of operators.

Personnel

1. It is essential that there is the closest cooperation between key personnel and those involved with computer systems. Persons in responsible positions should have the appropriate training for the management and use of systems within their field of responsibility which utilizes computers. This should include ensuring that appropriate expertise is available and used to provide advice on aspects of design, validation, installation and operation of computerized system.

Validation

2. The extent of validation necessary will depend on a number of factors including the use to which the system is to be put, whether the validation is to be prospective or retrospective and whether or not novel elements are incorporated. Validation should be considered as part of the complete life cycle of a computer system. This cycle includes the stages of planning, specification, programming, testing, commissioning, documentation, operation, monitoring and modifying.

System

3. Attention should be paid to the siting of equipment in suitable conditions where extraneous factors cannot interfere with the system.

4. A written detailed description of the system should be produced (including diagrams as appropriate) and kept up to date. It should describe the principles, objectives, security measures and scope of the system and the main features of the way in which the computer is used and how it interacts with other systems and procedures.

5. The software is a critical component of a computerized system. The user of such software should take all reasonable steps to ensure that it has been produced in accordance with a system of Quality Assurance.

6. The system should include, where appropriate, built-in checks of the correct entry and processing of data.

7. Before a system using a computer is brought into use, it should be thoroughly tested and confirmed as being capable of achieving the desired results. If a manual system is being replaced, the two should be run in parallel for a time, as a part of this testing and validation.

8. Data should only be entered or amended by persons authorized to do so. Suitable methods of deterring unauthorized entry of data include the use of keys, pass cards, personal codes and restricted access to computer terminals. There should be a defined procedure for the issue, cancellation, and alteration of authorization to enter and amend data, including the changing of personal passwords. Consideration should be given to systems allowing for recording of attempts to access by unauthorized persons.

9. When critical data are being entered manually (for example the weight and batch number of an ingredient during dispensing), there should be an additional check on the accuracy of the record which is made. This check may be done by a second operator or by validated electronic means.

10. The system should record the identity of operators entering or confirming critical data. Authority to amend entered data should be restricted to nominated persons. Any alteration to an entry of critical data should be authorized and recorded with the reason for the change. Consideration should be given to building into the system the creation of a complete record of all entries and amendments (an "audit trail").

11. Alterations to a system or to a computer program should only be made in accordance with a defined procedure which should include provision for validating, checking, approving and implementing the change. Such an alteration should only be implemented with the agreement of the person responsible for the part of the system concerned, and the alteration should be recorded. Every significant modification should be validated.

12. For quality auditing purposes, it should be possible to obtain clear printed copies of electronically stored data.

13. Data should be secured by physical or electronic means against wilful or accidental damage, in accordance with item 4.9. of the Guide. Stored data should be checked for accessibility, durability and accuracy. If changes are proposed to the computer equipment or its programs, the above mentioned checks should be performed at a frequency appropriate to the storage medium being used.

14. Data should be protected by backing-up at regular intervals. Back-up data should be stored as long as necessary at a separate and secure location.

15. There should be available adequate alternative arrangements for systems which need to be operated in the event of a breakdown. The time required to bring the alternative arrangements into use should be related to the possible urgency of the need to use them. For example, information required to effect a recall must be available at short notice.

16. The procedures to be followed if the system fails or breaks down should be defined and validated. Any failures and remedial action taken should be recorded.

17. A procedure should be established to record and analyze errors and to enable corrective action to be taken.

18. When outside agencies are used to provide a computer service, there should be a formal agreement including a clear statement of the responsibilities of that outside agency (see Chapter 7).

19. When the release of batches for sale or supply is carried out using a computerized system, the system should allow for only a Qualified Person to release the batches and it should clearly identify and record the person releasing the batches.

ANNEX 12 USE OF IONIZING RADIATION IN THE MANUFACTURE OF MEDICINAL PRODUCTS

Note

The holder of, or applicant for, a marketing authorization for a product which includes irradiation as part of its processing should also refer to the note produced by the Committee for Proprietary Medicinal Products giving guidance on "Ionizing radiation in the manufacture of medicinal products".

Introduction

Ionizing radiation may be used during the manufacturing process for various purposes including the reduction of bioburden and the sterilization of starting materials, packaging components or products and the treatment of blood products.

There are two types of irradiation process: Gamma Irradiation from a radioactive source and high energy Electron Irradiation (Beta radiation) from an accelerator.

Gamma Irradiation: two different processing modes may be employed:

(i) Batch mode: the product is arranged at fixed locations around the radiation source and cannot be loaded or unloaded while the radiation source is exposed.

(ii) Continuous mode: an automatic system conveys the products into the radiation cell, past the exposed radiation source along a defined path and at an appropriate speed, and out of the cell.

Electron Irradiation: the product is conveyed past a continuous or pulsed beam of high energy electrons (Beta radiation) which is scanned back and forth across the product pathway.

Responsibilities

1. Treatment by irradiation may be carried out by the pharmaceutical manufacturer or by an operator of a radiation facility under contract (a "contract manufacturer"), both of whom must hold an appropriate manufacturing authorization.

2. The pharmaceutical manufacturer bears responsibility for the quality of the product including the attainment of the objective of irradiation. The contract operator of the radiation facility bears responsibility for ensuring that the dose of radiation required by the manufacturer is delivered to the irradiation container (i.e. the outermost container in which the products are irradiated).

3. The required dose including justified limits will be stated in the marketing authorization for the product.

Dosimetry

4. Dosimetry is defined as the measurement of the absorbed dose by the use of dosimeters. Both understanding and correct use of the technique is essential for the validation, commissioning and control of the process.

5. The calibration of each batch of routine dosimeters should be traceable to a national or international standard. The period of validity of the calibration should be stated, justified and adhered to.

6. The same instrument should normally be used to establish the calibration curve of the routine dosimeters and to measure the change in their absorbance after irradiation. If a different instrument is used, the absolute absorbance of each instrument should be established.

7. Depending on the type of dosimeter used, due account should be taken of possible causes of inaccuracy including the change in moisture content, change in temperature, time elapsed between irradiation and measurement, and the dose rate.

8. The wavelength of the instrument used to measure the change in absorbance of dosimeters and the instrument used to measure their thickness should be subject to regular checks of calibration at intervals established on the basis of stability, purpose and usage.

Validation of the process

9. Validation is the action of proving that the process, i.e. the delivery of the intended absorbed dose to the product, will achieve the expected results. The requirements for validation are given more fully in the note for guidance on "the use of ionizing radiation in the manufacture of medicinal products".

10. Validation should include dose mapping to establish the distribution of absorbed dose within the irradiation container when packed with product in a defined configuration.

11. An irradiation process specification should include at least the following:
    (a) details of the packaging of the product;
    (b) the loading pattern(s) of product within the irradiation container. Particular care needs to be taken, when a mixture of products is allowed in the irradiation container, that there is no underdosing of dense product or shadowing of other products by dense product. Each mixed product arrangement must be specified and validated;
    (c) the loading pattern of irradiation containers around the source (batch mode) or the pathway through the cell (continuous mode);
    (d) maximum and minimum limits of absorbed dose to the product [and associated routine dosimetry];

(e) maximum and minimum limits of absorbed dose to the irradiation container and associated routine dosimetry to monitor this absorbed dose;
(f) other process parameters, including dose rate, maximum time of exposure, number of exposures, etc.

When irradiation is supplied under contract at least parts (d) and (e) of the irradiation process specification should form part of that contract.

Commissioning of the plant

General

12. Commissioning is the exercise of obtaining and documenting evidence that the irradiation plant will perform consistently within predetermined limits when operated according to the process specification. In the context of this annex, predetermined limits are the maximum and minimum doses designed to be absorbed by the irradiation container. It must not be possible for variations to occur in the operation of the plant which give a dose to the container outside these limits without the knowledge of the operator.

13. Commissioning should include the following elements:
(a) Design;
(b) Dose mapping;
(c) Documentation;
(d) Requirement for re-commissioning.

Gamma Irradiators

14. *Design*

The absorbed dose received by a particular part of an irradiation container at any specific point in the irradiator depends primarily on the following factors:
(a) the activity and geometry of the source;
(b) the distance from source to container;
(c) The duration of irradiation controlled by the timer setting or conveyor speed;
(d) The composition and density of material, including other products, between the source and the particular part of the container.

15. The total absorbed dose will in addition depend on the path of containers through a continuous irradiator or the loading pattern in a batch irradiator, and on the number of exposure cycles.

16. For a continuous irradiator with a fixed path or a batch irradiator with a fixed loading pattern, and with a given source strength and type of product, the key plant parameter control led by the operator is conveyor speed or timer setting.

17. *Dose Mapping*

For the dose mapping procedure, the irradiator should be filled with irradiation containers packed with dummy products or a representative product of uniform density. Dosimeters should be placed throughout a minimum of three loaded irradiation containers which are passed through the irradiator, surrounded by similar containers or dummy products. If the product is not uniformly packed, dosimeters should be placed in a larger number of containers.

18. The positioning of dosimeters will depend on the size of the irradiation container. For example, for containers up to 1 x 1 x 0.5 m, a three-dimensional 20 cm grid throughout the container including the outside surfaces might be suitable. If the expected positions of the minimum and maximum dose are known from a previous irradiator performance characterization, some dosimeters could be removed from regions of average dose and replaced to form a 10 cm grid in the regions of extreme dose.

19. The results of this procedure will give minimum and maximum absorbed doses in the product and on the container surface for a given set of plant parameters, product density and loading pattern.

20. Ideally, reference dosimeters should be used for the dose mapping exercise because of their greater precision. Routine dosimeters are permissible but it is advisable to place reference dosimeters beside them at the expected positions of minimum and maximum dose and at the routine monitoring position in each of the replicate irradiation containers. The observed values of dose will have an associated random uncertainty which can be estimated from the variations in replicate measurements.

21. The minimum observed dose, as measured by the routine dosimeters, necessary to ensure that all irradiation containers receive the minimum required dose will be set in the knowledge of the random variability of the routine dosimeters used.

22. Irradiator parameters should be kept constant, monitored and recorded during dose mapping. The records, together with the dosimetry results and all other records generated, should be retained.

Electron Beam Irradiators

23. *Design*

The absorbed dose received by a particular portion of an irradiated product depends primarily on the following factors:

(a) the characteristics of the beam, which are: electron energy, average beam current, scan width and scan uniformity;

(b) the conveyor speed;

(c) the product composition and density;

(d) the composition, density and thickness of material between the output window and the particular portion of product;

(e) the output window to container distance.

24. Key parameters controlled by the operator are the characteristics of the beam and the conveyor speed.

25. *Dose Mapping*

For the dose mapping procedure, dosimeters should be placed between layers of homogeneous absorber sheets making up a dummy product, or between layers of representative products of uniform density, such that at least ten measurements can be made within the maximum range of the electrons. Reference should also be made to sections 18 to 21.

26. Irradiator parameters should be kept constant, monitored and recorded during dose mapping. The records, together with the dosimetry results and all other records generated, should be retained.

Re-commissioning

27. Commissioning should be repeated if there is a change to the process or the irradiator which could affect the dose distribution to the irradiation container (e.g. change of source pencils). The extent to re-commissioning depends on the extent of the change in the irradiator or the load that has taken place. If in doubt, re-commission.

Premises

28. Premises should be designed and operated to segregate irradiated from non-irradiated containers to avoid their cross-contamination. Where materials are handled within closed irradiation containers, it may not be necessary to segregate pharmaceutical from non-pharmaceutical materials, provided there is no risk of the former being contaminated by the latter.

Any possibility of contamination of the products by radionuclide from the source must be excluded.

Processing

29. Irradiation containers should be packed in accordance with the specified loading pattern(s) established during validation.

30. During the process, the radiation dose to the irradiation containers should be monitored using validated dosimetry procedures. The relationship between this dose and

the dose absorbed by the product inside the container must have been established during process validation and plant commissioning.

31. Radiation indicators should be used as an aid to differentiating irradiated from non-irradiated containers. They should not be used as the sole means of differentiation or as an indication of satisfactory processing.

32. Processing of mixed loads of containers within the irradiation cell should only be done when it is known from commissioning trials or other evidence that the radiation dose received by individual containers remains within the limits specified.

33. When the required radiation dose is by design given during more than one exposure or passage through the plant, this should be with the agreement of the holder of the marketing authorization and occur within a predetermined time period. Unplanned interruptions during irradiation should be notified to the holder of the marketing authorization if this extends the irradiation process beyond a previously agreed period.

34. Non-irradiated products must be segregated from irradiated products at all times. Methods of doing this include the use of radiation indicators (31.) and appropriate design of premises (28.).

Gamma Irradiators

35. For continuous processing modes, dosimeters should be placed so that at least two are exposed in the irradiation at all times.

36. For batch modes, at least two dosimeters should be exposed in positions related to the minimum dose position.

37. For continuous process modes, there should be a positive indication of the correct position of the source and an interlock between source position and conveyor movement. Conveyor speed should be monitored continuously and recorded.

38. For batch process modes source movement and exposure times for each batch should be monitored and recorded.

39. For a given desired dose, the timer setting or conveyor speed requires adjustment for source decay and source additions. The period of validity of the setting or speed should be recorded and adhered to.

Electron Beam Irradiators

40. A dosimeter should be placed on every container.

41. There should be continuous recording of average beam current, electron energy, scan-width and conveyor speed. These variables, other than conveyor speed, need

to be controlled within the defined limits established during commissioning since they are liable to instantaneous change.

Documentation

42. The numbers of containers received, irradiated and dispatched should be reconciled with each other and with the associated documentation. Any discrepancy should be reported and resolved.

43. The irradiation plant operator should certify in writing the range of doses received by each irradiated container within a batch or delivery.

44. Process and control records for each irradiation batch should be checked and signed by a nominated responsible person and retained. The method and place of retention should be agreed between the plant operator and the holder of the marketing authorization.

45. The documentation associated with the validation and commissioning of the plant should be retained for one year after the expiry date or at least five years after the release of the last product processed by the plant, whichever is the longer.

Microbiological monitoring

46. Microbiological monitoring is the responsibility of the pharmaceutical manufacturer. It may include environmental monitoring where product is manufactured and pre-irradiation monitoring of the product as specified in the marketing authorization.

ANNEX 13 GOOD MANUFACTURING PRACTICE FOR INVESTIGATIONAL MEDICINAL PRODUCTS

Introduction

Medicinal products intended for research and development trials are not at present subject either to marketing or manufacturing Community legislation.

However, when adopting Directive 91/356/EEC on GMP for medicinal products for human use, it was agreed to include a "whereas" stating that Member States may require compliance with the principles of GMP during the manufacture of products intended for use in clinical trials. It was also suggested in a EC Discussion Paper (111/3044/91) in January 1991 that it is illogical for experimental products not to be subject to the controls which would apply to the formulations of which they are the prototypes and most of the comments received from interested parties were in line with this suggestion.

Therefore it was agreed to prepare this annex to the Community Guide to Good Manufacturing Practice so that both those Member States instituting controls voluntarily and manufacturers of investigational products would have a reference point to enable common standards to evolve in all Member States.

This annex will be reviewed in the light of any development of Community legislation in the area of clinical investigation.

Note

The principles and many of the detailed guidelines of Good manufacturing Practice for Medicinal Products (Volume IV of the series "The rules governing medicinal products in the European Community)" are relevant to the preparation of products for use in clinical trials.

This annex specifically address those practices which may be different for investigational products, which are usually not manufactured under a set routine, and with possibly incomplete characterisation of the product at initial stages of clinical development. They also include guidance on ordering, shipping, and returning clinical supplies, which are at the interface with the Community Note for Guidance on Good Clinical Practice for trials on medicinal products.

Glossary

Clinical trial

Any systematic study of medicinal products in human subjects whether in patients or healthy volunteers in. order to discover or verify the effects of and/or identify any adverse reaction to investigational medicinal products, and/or to study their absorption, distribution, metabolism and excretion in order to ascertain the efficacy and safety of the products.

Investigational product

A pharmaceutical form of an active ingredient or placebo being tested or used as a reference in a clinical trial (including a product with a marketing authorisation when used or assembled other than as authorised).

Investigator

Person responsible for the practical performance of a trial and for the integrity, health and welfare of the subjects during the trial.

Order

Instruction to process, package and/or ship a certain number of units of investigational product.

Product specification file

Reference file containing all the information necessary to draft the detailed written instructions on processing, packaging, quality control testing, batch release and shipping.

Shipping/dispatch

The operation of assembly, packaging for shipment, and sending of ordered medicinal products for clinical trials.

Sponsor

Individual or organisation which takes responsibility for the initiation, management and/or financing of a clinical trial.

Quality Management

1. Some of the production processes of investigational products which have no marketing authorisation may not be validated to the extent necessary for a routine production operation. The product specifications and manufacturing instructions may vary during development. This increased complexity in manufacturing operations requires a highly effective system of Quality Assurance.

2. The Quality Assurance System, designed, set up and verified by the manufacturer, should be described in writing, taking into account the GMP principles applied to investigational products.

3. Packaging and labelling operations are often performed after the release of the bulk product and in accordance with specific requirements of different trials. These operations are of paramount importance for the integrity of clinical trials. In this respect, self inspection or independent Quality Assurance audits, as referred to in the Note for Guidance on Good Clinical Practice and in 9.2 of the Guide to GMP are an integral part of the Quality Assurance system.

Personnel

4. Although it is likely that the number of staff involved will be small, there should be separate people responsible for production and quality control. All production operations should be carried out under control of a clearly identified responsible person and personnel involved in quality control testing need to be extra vigilant.

Premises and Equipment

5. During manufacture of investigational products, it may be that different products are handled in the same premises and at the same time, and this reinforces the need to eliminate all risks of contamination, including cross-contamination, by using appropriate procedures.

6. For the production of the particular products referred to in paragraph 3.6 of the Guide to GMP, campaign working may be acceptable in place of dedicated and self-contained facilities. Because the toxicity of the materials may not be fully known, cleaning is of particular importance; account should be taken of the solubility of the product and of excipients in various cleaning solvents.

7. For sterile products, there should be no reduction in the degree of validation of sterilising equipment. Validation of aseptic processes presents special problems when the batch size is small; in these cases the number of units filled may be the maximum number filled in production. Filling and sealing is often a hand operation presenting great challenges to sterility so enhanced attention should be given to environmental monitoring.

Documentation

8. Specifications (for starting materials, primary packaging materials, intermediate and bulk products and finished products), manufacturing formulae and processing and packaging instructions may be changed frequently as a result of new experience.

Each new version should take into account the latest data and should refer to the previous version so that traceability is ensured. Rationales for changes should be recorded.

9. It may not be necessary to produce Master Formula and Processing Instructions, but for every manufacturing operation or supply there should be clear and adequate written instructions and written records. Records are particularly important for the preparation of the final version of the documents to be used in routine manufacture.

10. Batch manufacturing records should be retained for at least two years after completion of the clinical trial.

Order

11. The order may request the processing and/or packaging of a certain number of units and/or their shipping. It may only be given by the sponsor to the manufacturer of an investigational products. It should be in writing (though it may be transmitted by electronic means), and precise enough to avoid any ambiguity, it should be formally authorised and it should refer to the approved Product Specification File.

Product Specification File

12. All the information necessary to draft the detailed written instructions on processing, packaging, quality control testing, batch release, storage conditions and/or shipping should be kept together in a Product Specification File. This Product Specification File should be continuously updated, ensuring appropriate traceability to the previous versions.

Specifications

13. Specifications may be subject to change as development of the product progresses. Changes should however be carried out according to a written procedure, authorised by a responsible person and clearly recorded. Specifications should be based on all available scientific data, current state-of-the-art, technology used, and the regulatory and pharmacopoeial requirements.

Manufacturing Formulae and Processing Instructions

14. They may be changed in the light of experience but allowance must be made for any possible repercussions on stability and, above all, on bio-equivalence between

batches of finished products. Changes should however be carried out according to a written procedure, authorised by a responsible person and clearly recorded.

Packaging Instructions

15. Packaging and labelling of investigational products are likely to be more complex and more liable to errors (which are also harder to detect) than with licensed products when "blinded" labels are used. Supervision procedures such as label reconciliation, line clearance, etc and the independent checks by quality control staff should accordingly be intensified.

16. Packaging instructions are based on the order. Contrary to what happens with large-scale manufacturing of licensed medicinal products, batches of investigational medicinal products may be subdivided into different packaging batches and packaged in several operations over a period of time.

17. The number of units to package should be specified prior to the start of the packaging operations, considering also the number of units necessary for carrying out quality controls and the number of samples to be kept. A reconciliation should take place at the end of the packaging and labelling process.

Labelling instructions

18. Labels should include:
    - the name of the sponsor
    - a trial reference number
    - the batch number
    - the patient identification number
    - the storage conditions
    - the expiry date in month/year or a re-test date

    Additional information may be displayed according to the order. When necessary for blinding purposes, the batch number may be provided separately (see also "blinding operations"). A copy of each type of label should be kept in the batch packaging record.

Manufacturing and packaging batch records

19. Manufacturing and packaging batch records should be kept in sufficient detail for the sequence of operations to be accurately traced back. These records should contain any relevant remarks which enhance existing knowledge of the product and

allow improvements of the manufacturing operations and justify the procedures used.

Production

Starting materials

20. The consistency of production may be influenced by quality of the starting materials. Their physical and chemical properties should therefore be defined, documented in their specifications and controlled. Specifications for active ingredients should be as comprehensive as possible, given the current state of knowledge. Specifications for both active and non-active ingredients should be periodically re-assessed.

21. Detailed information on the quality of active and nonactive ingredients should be available in order to recognise and, as necessary, allow for any variation of the production.

Manufacturing operations

22. During the development phase, validated procedures may not always be available, which makes it difficult to know in advance the critical parameters and the in-process controls that would help to control these parameters. In these cases, provisional production parameters and in-process controls may usually be deduced from experience with analogs. Careful consideration by key personnel is called for in order to formulate the necessary instructions and to adapt them continuously to the experience gained in production.

23. Calculation of yields is an essential part of the control of the manufacturing operations. Actual and theoretical yields should be reconciled and any abnormal discrepancy investigated.

24. Assurance of sterility for sterile medicinal products should be no less than for licensed products. Cleaning procedures should be very stringent and designed in the light of the incomplete knowledge of the toxicity of the investigational product. Where processes such as mixing have not been validated, additional quality control testing may be necessary.

Principles applicable to comparator drug

25. In studies whereby an investigational product is compared with a marketed product, attention should be paid to ensure the integrity and quality of the comparator product (final dosage form, packaging materials, storage conditions, etc). If significant changes are to be made to the product, data should be available (eg stability, com-

parative dissolution) to prove that these changes do not influence the original quality characteristics of the product.

Randomisation code

26. Procedures should describe the generation, distribution, handling and retention of any randomisation code used for packaging investigational products.

Blinding operations

27. A coding system should be implemented to allow for a proper identification of the 'blinded' products. The code, together with the randomisation code and randomisation list must allow proper identification of the product, including any necessary Traceability to the codes and batch number of the product before the blinding operation.

28. The release of 'blinded' products should include a formal check on the similarity in appearance and any other required characteristics between the different products being compared.

29. Samples of blinded investigational products should be retained.

Quality Control

30. As processes may not be standardised or fully validated, end product testing takes on more importance to ensure that each batch meets its specification.

31. Product release is often carried out in two stages, before and after final packaging:
    - bulk product assessment: it should cover all relevant factors, including production conditions, results of in-process testing, a review of manufacturing documentation and compliance with the Product Specification File and the Order;
    - finished product assessment: it should cover, in addition to the bulk product assessment, all relevant factors, including packaging conditions, results of in-process testing, a review of packaging documentation and compliance with the Product Specification File and the Order.

32. Quality control should especially pay attention to the compliance with specifications which bear on the efficacy of medicinal products, namely:
    - accuracy of the therapeutic or unitary dose: homogeneity, content uniformity;
    - release of active ingredients: solubility, partition coefficient, dissolution time, etc.
    - estimation of stability, if necessary in accelerated conditions, determination of the preliminary storage conditions and shelf-life of the product.

When necessary, Quality Control should also verify the similarity in appearance, smell and taste of "blinded" medicinal products.

33. Samples of each batch of product should be retained in the primary container used for the study or in a suitable bulk container for at least one year beyond the final shelf-life. If the sample is not stored in the pack used for the study, stability data should be available to justify the shelf-life in the pack used.

Contract Manufacture and Analysis

34. The contract must clearly state, among other provisions, the use of the medicinal products in clinical trials. Cooperation between the contracting parties should be very close.

Complaints

35. The conclusions of any investigation carried out in relation to a complaint should be discussed between the manufacturer and the sponsor (if different) or between the persons responsible for manufacture and those responsible for the relevant clinical trial in order to assess any potential impact on the trial and on the product development.

Recalls

36. Recall procedures are important. They should be understood by the sponsor, investigator and monitor in addition to the person(s) responsible for recalls, as described in the Chapter 8 of the guide.

Shipping – Returns – Destruction

37. Shipping, return and destruction of unused products should be carried out according to written procedures.

Shipping

38. Shipping of investigational products is conducted according to orders given by the sponsor in the shipping order.

39. A shipment is sent to an investigator only after a two step release procedure: the release of the product after quality control ('technical green light') and the authorisa-

tion to use the product, given by the sponsor ('regulatory green light'). Both releases should be recorded.

40. The packaging must ensure that the medicinal product remains in good condition during transport and storage at intermediate destinations. Any opening or tampering of the outer packaging during transport should be readily discernible.

41. The sponsor should ensure that the shipment is to be received and acknowledged by the right addressee.

42. A detailed inventory of the shipments made by the manufacturer should be maintained. It should particularly mention the addressees' identification.

Returns

43. Investigational products should be returned on agreed conditions defined by the sponsor, specified in written procedures, and approved by authorised staff members.

44. Returned investigational products should be clearly identified and stored in a dedicated area. Inventory records of the returned medicinal products should be kept.

Destruction

45. The Sponsor is responsible for the destruction of unused investigational products. Investigational products should therefore not be destroyed by the manufacturer without prior authorisation by the Sponsor.

46. Recording of destruction operations should be carried out in such a manner that all operations may be accounted for. The records should be kept by the Sponsor.

47. If the manufacturer is requested to destroy the products, he should deliver a certificate of destruction or a receipt for destruction to the Sponsor. These documents should clearly identify the batches involved and the actual quantities destroyed.

ANNEX 14 MANUFACTURE OF PRODUCTS DERIVED FROM HUMAN BLOOD OR HUMAN PLASMA

Principle

Medicinal products derived from human blood or plasma have certain special features arising from the biological nature of the source material. For example, disease-transmitting agents, especially viruses, may contaminate the source material. The prevention of the transmission of viruses by these products relies therefore on the control of source materials and their origin as well as on the subsequent manufacturing procedures, including virus removal and inactivation.

Since the quality of the final products is affected by all the steps in their manufacture, including the collection of blood or plasma, the collection of blood or plasma intended for the manufacture of derivatives should be considered as part of the manufacturing process and it should therefore be done in accordance with an appropriate system of Quality Assurance and the current Good Manufacturing Practice.

Note

The general chapters of the guide to GMP apply to products derived from human blood or plasma, unless otherwise stated. Some of the annexes may also -apply, e.g. manufacture of sterile medicinal products, use of ionizing radiation in the manufacture of medicinal products and the annex on biological medicinal products.

By virtue of Directive 89/381/EEC, the measures necessary to prevent the transmission of infectious diseases shall comprise those currently recommended by the Council of Europe (see "Guide to the preparation, use and quality assurance of blood components", Council of Europe Press, ISBN 92-871-1808-4) and by the World Health Organization (see thirty-ninth report of the WHO Expert Committee on Biological Standardization, WHO Technical Report Series 786, 1989).

This annex should also be read in conjunction with the guidelines adopted by the CPMP, in particular "Medicinal products derived from human blood and plasma" and "Validation of virus removal and inactivation procedures" (Vol III addendum 2 of the series "The rules governing medicinal products in the European Community).

As several provisions of this annex apply equally to plasma, to products derived from plasma, to cellular components and to whole blood, an additional paragraph relating to cellular components and whole blood only has been added for the convenience of those competent authorities wishing to control these components. It should however be noted that these components are presently not included in the scope of EC pharmaceutical legislation.

The manufacture of medicinal products derived from placental blood, which are manufactured and used in some Member States, is not the subject of this annex. There are therefore no special provisions in this annex for the manufacture of these medicinal products; nevertheless, all the relevant provisions of the guide to GMP apply to their manufacture.

Quality Management

1. Quality Assurance should cover all aspects of manufacture, starting with the donor, blood bags, anticoagulant solutions and including collection, storage, transportation, processing, quality control and delivery of the finished product(*).

2. Only blood or plasma collected in centres subject to inspection and approved by a competent authority should be processed.

3. Full testing of qualitative and quantitative requirements mentioned in the specifications for starting materials is not normally performed on intermediate fractions of blood products. Control reports issued by the producer of the intermediate material, including plasma, will suffice, provided that the producer is a manufacturer authorized in accordance with Community legislation, is regularly inspected and there is a history of reliability and consistency.

4. Results of the controls carried out on the accepted donors should be part of the quality documentation of the collecting centre and should be available to the manufacturer.

Premises and equipment

5. Blood collection may be done on a campaign basis, i.e. in a room used at the time exclusively for that purpose, or in dedicated facilities. Dedicated facilities should be used for blood and plasma processing, but are not required for packaging operations.

6. In order to prevent cross-contamination, premises and equipment used for manufacturing operations using products which have undergone a process of virus removal or inactivation should be dedicated and distinct from those used for non-treated products.

Blood collection

7. The method used to disinfect the skin of the donor should be clearly defined and shown to be effective. Adherence to that method should then be maintained.

(*) It should be noted that, although desirable, the normal organizational chart of a manufacturing plant, with a full-time Head of Production Department, a Head of the Quality Control Department and the Qualified Person, as described in the Chapter 2 of the Guide, is not necessarily applicable for blood collection and plasmapheresis centres.

8. The identity of each donor should be recorded during selection and confirmed before venepuncture. A third identification, preferably by a signature check, will be necessary during manual apheresis, where components are being returned after disconnection.

9. Special attention should be given to the correct labelling and identification (code number) of donor samples.

10. There should be a system in place which enables the path taken by each donation to be traced, both forward from the donor [and the blood bag] and back from the finished product, including the identification of the customer (hospital or health care professional). It is normally the responsibility of this customer to identify the recipient.

11. Post-collection measures: A standard operating procedure describing the mutual information system between the blood collection centre and the manufacturing or fractionation centre should be set up so that they can inform each other if:
    - it is found subsequent to donation that the donor did not meet the current donor health criteria;
    - it is discovered that testing for viral markers has not been carried out according to agreed procedures;
    - the donor seroconverts or develops an infectious disease as a result of a transmissible agent (HBV, HCV and other non-A, non-B, non-C hepatitis viruses, HIV 1 and 2 and other viruses, in the light of current knowledge);
    - the recipient develops post transfusion infection which implicates or can be traced back to the donor.

    In these cases, a re-assessment of the batch documentation and re-control of finished products should always be carried out. The need for withdrawal of the given batch should be carefully considered, taking into consideration criteria such as the disease, the type of seroconversions, the size of the pool, the time period between donation and seroconversion, and the nature of the product and its manufacturing method.

Production and Quality Control

12. The specified storage temperatures of blood, plasma and intermediate products during transportation from collection centres to manufacturers or between different manufacturing sites should be checked and validated. The same applies to delivery of these products.

13 Before any blood and plasma donations, or any product derived there from, are released for issue and/or fractionation, they should be tested and found non reactive for the following markers of specific disease-transmitting agents:
    - HBsAg, using a validated and sensitive ELISA or RIA test;

- antibodies to HIV 1 and HIV 2;
- antibodies to HCV;
- syphilis antibodies(*)

Testing requirements for other viruses should be considered in the light of knowledge emerging as to infectious agents and the availability of appropriate test methods.

14. Some manufacturing operations may place the product at risk and consideration should be given to the following factors:
    - bacteria may be introduced by inappropriate handling or from a contaminated environment and may lead to the accumulation of pyrogens;
    - viruses may be introduced by reagents during manufacture (enzymes from tissues extracts, such as pepsin or thrombin, or monoclonal antibodies used for affinity chromatography);
    - the methods of manufacture may introduce chemical contaminants such as enzymes, pepsin, solvents, detergents and antibodies or other ligands from chromatography.

15. The efficacy of cleaning procedures and sterile docking should be regularly controlled and validated.

16. The labels on single units of plasma stored before pooling and fractionation should bear at least the identification number of the donation, the name and address of the plasma collection centre, the batch number of the container, the storage temperature, the total volume or weight of the plasma, the quantity and type of the anticoagulant used and the date of collection and/or separation.

17. In order to minimise the microbiological contamination of plasma or the introduction of foreign material, the pooling and thawing of plasma should be performed at least in a grade D clean area and face masks and gloves should be worn. Methods used for opening bags, pooling and thawing should be regularly monitored.

18. Products which have undergone a process of virus removal or inactivation should be clearly differentiated from those which have not.

19. Validation of methods used for virus removal or virus inactivation should not be conducted in the production facilities in order not to put the routine manufacture at any risk of contamination with the viruses used for validation.

Fractionation/purification Procedures:

(a) Precipitation methods

20. Physical methods: cryoprecipitation is often used as the initial step for the production of Factor VIII and fibrinogen. It has no impact on the viral safety of such prod-

(*) this test is not required in Denmark.

ucts. Subsequent purification techniques, such as precipitation by agents other than ethanol or chromatographic separation as well as procedures for viral inactivation are used to obtain the finished products. Cryoprecipitate-depleted plasma can be used for the separation of other coagulation factors or plasma protein solutions.

21. Physical/chemical methods: among these methods, the ethanol fractionation procedures derived from the Cohn method are the most widely used, at least for albumin and immunoglobulins. They commonly incorporate several steps, in each of which compliance with specific requirements is decisive for product quality; under proper conditions, some of these steps may also contribute to the effective reduction of potential viral contaminants. Therefore, there should be clear instructions for ethanol and protein concentration, with data on acceptable tolerances as well as the means of controlling them.

22. Appropriate instructions should also exist for methods relying on other chemical agents such as ethylacridinlactate, methanol, ammonium sulphate, polyethylene glycol, cationic detergents, which are sometimes used in the preparation of certain plasma derivatives, as a rule in combination with other purification procedures. Some of these substances may have an impact on viral safety.

(b) Solid phase separation and filtration methods

23. Three basic types of procedures play an increasing role in the processing of plasma derivatives, as a rule in combination with precipitation procedures and often with each other:
    - gel filtration, mainly used for desalination or separation of components of significantly different sizes;
    - ion exchange and hydrophobic interaction chromatography;
    - affinity chromatography based on specific interactions with immunological or other receptors immobilized on the matrix.

    The selectivity of these procedures and the yields depend critically on the quality of the material as well as on factors such as the capacity of the column, the nature and concentration of proteins in the product, the ionic strength and pH of buffers, as well as the flow rate and temperature. Therefore, all appropriate data, including acceptable tolerances should be described in specifications and the control data should be recorded in the batch dossier.

24. Several other compounds such as charcoal, bentonite, and colloidal silica are sometimes used for removing various impurities such as pigments, lipoproteins, etc. Details of the characteristics of these compounds and their decontamination should be described in their specifications and the operating conditions should be detailed in procedures.

25. Directions for the storing of columns, the preservation and elution of preservatives and the methods of regeneration should also be given in procedures. Procedures used for clarification and sterile, dia-or ultra- filtration should also be available.

Retention of samples

26. Samples of each pool of plasma should be stored under suitable conditions for at least one year after the expiry date of the finished product with the longest shelf-life.

Cellular products and whole blood.

27. Quality monitoring should be carried out in such a way that major deviations of quality specifications are detected.
28. A visual inspection for the absence of haemolysis and aggregation should be carried out before red cells products or whole blood are issued. Platelet concentrates should be checked for the swirling effect.
29. Cells, platelets and whole blood which have been returned unused should normally not be reissued (see point 5.65 of the guide).

GLOSSARY

Definitions given below apply to the words as used in this guide. They may have different meanings in other contexts. An additional glossary of terms relating to clinical trials is provided in Annex 13, good manufacturing practice for investigational products.

Air-lock

An enclosed space with two or more doors, and which is interposed between two or more rooms, e.g. of differing class of cleanliness, for the purpose of controlling the air-flow between those rooms when they need to be entered. An air-lock is designed for and used by either people or goods.

Batch (or lot)

A defined quantity of starting material, packaging material or product processed in one process or series of processes so that it could be expected to be homogeneous.

Note: To complete certain stages of manufacture, it may be necessary to divide a batch into a number of subbatches, which are later brought together to form a final homogeneous batch. In the case of continuous manufacture, the batch must correspond to a defined fraction of the production, characterized by its intended homogeneity.

For control of the finished product, the following definition has been given in Directive 75/318/EEC: 'For the control of the finished product, a batch of a proprietary medicinal product comprises all the units of a pharmaceutical form which are made from the same initial mass of material and have undergone a single series of manufacturing operations or a single sterilization operation or, in the case of a continuous production process, all the units manufactured in a given period of time'.

Batch number (or lot number)

A distinctive combination of numbers and/or letters which specifically identifies a batch.

Biogenerator

A contained system, such as a fermenter, into which biological agents are introduced along with other materials so as to effect their multiplication or their production of other substances by reaction with the other materials. Biogenerators are generally fitted with devices for regulation, control, connection, material addition and material withdrawal.

Biological Agents

Microorganisms, including genetically engineered microorganisms, cell cultures and endoparasites, whether pathogenic or not.

Bulk product

Any product which has completed all processing stages up to, but not including, final packaging.

Calibration

The set of operations which establish, under specified conditions, the relationship between values indicated by a measuring instrument or measuring system, or values represented by a material measure, and the corresponding known values of a reference standard.

Cell bank

Cell bank system: A cell bank system is a system whereby successive batches of a product are manufactured by culture in cells derived from the same master cell bank (fully characterised for identity and absence of contamination). A number of containers from the master cell bank are used to prepare a working cell bank. The cell bank system is validated for a passage level or number of population doublings beyond that achieved during routine production.

Master cell bank: A culture of [fully characterized] cells distributed into containers in a single operation, processed together in such a manner as to ensure uniformity and stored in such a manner as to ensure stability. A master cell bank is usually stored at - 70°C or lower.

Working cell bank: A culture of cells derived from the master cell bank and intended for use in the preparation of production cell cultures. The working cell bank is usually stored at –70°C or lower.

Cell culture

The result from the in-vitro growth of cells isolated from multicellular organisms.

Clean area

An area with defined environmental control of particulate and microbial contamination, constructed and used in such a way as to reduce the introduction, generation and retention of contaminants within the area.

Note: The different degrees of environmental control are defined in the Supplementary Guidelines for the Manufacture of sterile medicinal products.

Clean/contained area

An area constructed and operated in such a manner that will achieve the aims of both a clean area and a contained area at the same time.

Containment

The action of confining a biological agent or other entity within a defined space.

Primary containment: A system of containment which prevents the escape of a biological agent into the immediate working environment. It involves the use of closed containers or safety biological cabinets along with secure operating procedures.

Secondary containment: A system of containment which prevents the escape of a biological agent into the external environment or into other working areas. It involves the use of rooms with specially designed air handling, the existence of airlocks and/or sterilizers for the exit of materials and secure operating procedures. In many cases it may add to the effectiveness of primary containment.

Contained area

An area constructed and operated in such a manner (and equipped with appropriate air handling and filtration) so as to prevent contamination of the external environment by biological agents from within the area.

Controlled area

An area constructed and operated in such a manner that some attempt is made to control the introduction of potential contamination (an air supply approximating to grade D may be appropriate), and the consequences of accidental release of living organisms. The level of control exercized should reflect the nature of the organism employed in the process. At a minimum, the area should be maintained at a pressure negative to the immediate external environment and allow for the efficient removal of small quantities of airborne contaminants.

Computerized system

A system including the input of data, electronic processing and the output of information to be used either for reporting or automatic control.

Cross contamination

Contamination of a material or of a product with another material or product.

Crude plant (vegetable drug)

Fresh or dried medicinal plant or parts thereof.

Cryogenic vessel

A container designed to contain liquefied gas at extremely low temperature.

Cylinder

A container designed to contain gas at a high pressure.

Exotic organism

A biological agent where either the corresponding disease does not exist in a given country or geographical area, or where the disease is the subject of prophylactic measures or an eradication programme undertaken in the given country or geographical area.

Finished product

A medicinal product which has undergone all stages of production, including packaging in its final container.

Herbal medicinal product

Medicinal product containing, as active ingredients, exclusively plant material and/or vegetable drug preparations.

Infected

Contaminated with extraneous biological agents and therefore capable of spreading infection.

In-process control

Checks performed during production in order to monitor and if necessary to adjust the process to ensure that the product conforms its specification. The control of the environment or equipment may also be regarded as a part of in-process control.

Intermediate product

Partly processed material which must undergo further manufacturing steps before it becomes a bulk product.

Liquifiable gases

Those which, at the normal filling temperature and pressure, remain as a liquid in the cylinder.

Manifold

Equipment or apparatus designed to enable one or more gas containers to be filled simultaneously from the same source.

Manufacture

All operations of purchase of materials and products, Production, Quality Control, release, storage, distribution of medicinal products and the related controls.

Manufacturer

Holder of a Manufacturing Authorization as described in Article 16 of Directive 75/319/EEC.

Medicinal plant

Plant the whole or part of which is used for medicinal purpose.

Medicinal product

Any substance or combination of substances presented for treating or preventing disease in human beings or animals.

Any substance or combination of substances which may be administered to human beings or animals with a view to making a medical diagnosis or to restoring, correcting or modifying physiological functions in human beings or in animals is likewise considered a medicinal product.

Packaging

All operations, including filling and labelling, which a bulk product has to undergo in order to become a finished product.

Note: Sterile filling would not normally be regarded as part of packaging, the bulk product being the filled, but not finally packaged, primary containers.

Packaging material

Any material employed in the packaging of a medicinal product, excluding any outer packaging used for transportation or shipment. Packaging materials are referred to as primary or secondary according to whether or not they are intended to be in direct contact with the product.

Procedures

Description of the operations to be carried out, the precautions to be taken and measures to be applied directly or indirectly related to the manufacture of a medicinal product.

Production

All operations involved in the preparation of a medicinal product, from receipt of materials, through processing and packaging, to its completion as a finished product.

Qualification

Action of proving that any equipment works correctly and actually leads to the expected results. The word *validation* is sometimes widened to incorporate the concept of qualification.

Quality control

See Chapter 1.

Quarantine

The status of starting or packaging materials, intermediate, bulk or finished products isolated physically or by other effective means whilst awaiting a decision on their release or refusal.

Radiopharmaceutical

"Radiopharmaceutical" shall mean any medicinal product which, when ready for use, contains one or more radionuclides (radioactive isotopes) included for a medicinal purpose (Directive 89/343/EEC extending the scope of Directives 65/65/EEC and 75/319/EEC to radiopharmaceuticals and laying down additional provisions.

Reconciliation

A comparison, making due allowance for normal variation, between the amount of product or materials theoretically and actually produced or used.

Record

See Chapter 4.

Recovery

The introduction of all or part of previous batches of the required quality into another batch at a defined stage of manufacture.

Reprocessing

The reworking of all or part of a batch of product of an unacceptable quality from a defined stage of production so that its quality may be rendered acceptable by one or more additional operations.

Return

Sending back to the manufacturer or distributor of a medicinal product which may or may not present a quality defect.

Seed lot

Seed lot system: A seed lot system is a system according to which successive batches of a product are derived from the same master seed lot at a given passage level. For routine production, a working seed lot is prepared from the master seed lot. The final product is derived from the working seed lot and has not undergone more passages from the master seed lot than the vaccine shown in clinical studies to be satisfactory with respect to safety and efficacy. The origin and the passage history of the master seed lot and the working seed lot are recorded.

Master seed lot: A culture of a micro-organism distributed from a single bulk into containers in a single operation in such a manner as to ensure uniformity, to prevent contamination and to ensure stability. A master seed lot in liquid form is usually stored at or below –70°C. A freeze-dried master seed lot is stored at a temperature known to ensure stability.

Working seed lot: A culture of a micro-organism derived from the master seed lot and intended for use in production. Working seed lots are distributed into containers and stored as described above for master seed lots.

Specification

See Chapter 4.

Starting material

Any substance used in the production of a medicinal product, but excluding packaging materials.

Sterility

Sterility is the absence of living organisms. The conditions of the sterility test are given in the European Pharmacopoeia.

System

Is used in the sense of a regulated pattern of interacting activities and techniques which are united to form an organized whole.

Validation

Action of proving, in accordance with the principles of Good Manufacturing Practice, that any procedure, process, equipment, material, activity or system actually leads to the expected results (see also qualification).

SUBJECT INDEX

Locators indicate chapter and paragraph numbers. A = annex; Ch. = chapter; Gls. = glossary.

Aerosol Products for Inhalation A10
  General A10.1
  Premises & Equipment A10.2–A10.3
  Production & Quality Control A10.4–A10.9
  Air Filtration A1.1, A1. 24, A5. 11
Air Grades:
  Biological Products A2.6
  Immunological Veterinary Products A5.9
  Pressurized Aerosols for Inhalation A10.3
  Protective Clothing & A1.14–A1.15
  Sterile Products A1.3–A1.6, A3.4, A4.10
Air-locks A1.22–A1.23, A5.11 Gls.
Air Supply Systems 3.12, 5.19
  Biological Products A2.13–A2.14
  Immunological Veterinary Products A5.11–A5.12
  Radiopharmaceuticals A3.3–A3.5
  Sterile Products A1.24–A1.26
Air Vent Filters A2.17
Ancillary Areas 3.30–3.33
Animals:
  Housing & Care 3.33, A2.21–A2.22, A5.18, A5.28–A5.31
  Quality Control Testing 6.22, A2.21
Aseptic Processing A1.6, A2.13
Audit Trail A11.10
  Blood products A14.8, A14.10

Bacillus Anthracis A2.9
Backing-up, Electronic Data A11.14
Batch (Lot) Gls.
  Number Gls.
Batch Processing Mode, Gamma Irradiation A12, A12.36, A12.38
Batch Records:
  Blood donations A14.4, A14.8
  Clinical Trial Products A13.9–A13.10
  Immunological Veterinary Products A5.51
  Irradiated Products A12.44
  Packaging 4.18
  Processing 4.17
  Retention 6.8

Sterile Products A1.55, A1.72
BCG Vaccine A2.4, A2.8
Beta Irradiation, See Electron Beam Irradiation
Biogenerator Gls.
Biological Agents Gls.
Containment A5.7–A5.20
Contamination of Personnel A5.3–A5.5
Handling A5. 56
Biological Indicators A1.53, A1.55, A1.63, A1.70–A1.71
Biological Medicinal Products A2
Animal Quarters & Care A2.21–A2.22
Documentation A2.23–A2.24
Personnel A2.1–A2.5, A2.32
Premises & Equipment A2.6–A2.20
Production A2.25–A2.40
Quality Control A2.41–A2.44
Blending Procedures A2.36, A5. 46
Blinded Products for Clinical Trial A13.27 – A13.29
Blood Products A14
Collection A14.1 – A14.11
Fractional Procedures A14.20 – A14.25
Premises and Equipment A14.5 – A14.6
Production and QC A14.12 – A14.19
Quality Management A14.1 – A14.4
Bulk Products Gls.
Processing Operations 5.35–5.39
Receipt 5.6
Specifications 4.12, A2.24

Calibration 3.41, Gls.
Campaign Working 3.6, 5.19, A2.10, A4.5, A4.7, A13.6
Cell Banks A2.27–A2.33, A5.40–A5.45, Gls.
Cell Cultures A2, Gls.
Centrifugation A2.36, A5.46
Chemical Indicators A1.55
Chromatography Equipment A2.40
Clean Areas A1.1–A1.4, Gls.
Blood Products A14.17
Classification A1.3
Equipment A1.27–A1.31
Immunological Veterinary Products A5.8, A5.10–A5.20
Personnel A1.7–A1.16, A1.41
Premises A1.17–A1.26
Sanitation A1.32–A1.25

Transfer Operations A5.48–A5.54
See also Sterile Products
Clean/Contained Area Gls.
Cleaning:
Clean Area Clothing A1.16
Clean Areas A1.32–A1.35
Containers & Valves for Aerosols A10.6
Design of Premises & 3.9–3.11, A1.17–A1.21, A2.15
Equipment 3.36, 5.19, A2.15
Gas Equipment/Pipelines A6.15
Clinical Trial Products A13
Collection of Blood and Plasma A14.1 – A14.11
Closed Systems 5.19, A2.11
Clostridium Botulinum A2.9
Clostridium Tetani A2.9
Clothing 2.15, 5.19
Animal Quarters A2.22
Changing Facilities 3.31, A1. 22, A2.22, A5.11–A5.12
Clean Areas A1.1–A1.16
Contained/Clean Areas A5.4–A5.5
Commissioning, Radiation Treatment Plant A12.12–A12.27
Comparator Drug, Clinical Trials A13.25
Complaints 8.1–8.7
Clinical Trial Products A13.35
Computerized Systems 4.9, A11, Gls.
Personnel A11.1
Validation A11.2
Contained Areas Gls.
Premises A5.7, A5.10–A5.20
Transfer Operations A5.48–A5.54
Containers:
Cleanliness 5.48
Damaged 5.4
Immunological Veterinary Products A5.60–A5.63
Sample 6.13
Starting Materials 5.27, 5.30
Sterile Products A1.80–A1.82
Veterinary Medicinal Products A4.9
See also Cylinders; Packaging
Containment Gls.
Biological Products for Human Use A2.18
Immunological Veterinary Products A5.7–A5.8, A5.10–A5.20
Contamination, Prevention 3.1, 5.10, A1.36–A1.49, A5.5, A13.5
Continuous Cultures A2.44, A5.68

Continuous Processing Mode, Gamma Irradiation A12, A12.35, A12.37
Contracted-out Operations:
  Analysis 6.6, Ch. 7
  Clinical Trial Products A13.34
  Computerized Systems A11.18
  Manufacturing Ch. 7
  Radiation Treatment A12.1–A12.2, A12.11
Controlled Areas Gls.
Creams A9
  Premises & Equipment A9.1–A9.3
  Production A9.4–A9.9
  Sterile A1.5, A1.6
Cross-contamination Gls.
  Biological Products A2.7
  Blood Products A14.6
  Immunological Veterinary Products A5.5
  in Production 3.6, 5.18–5.20
  Veterinary Medicinal Products A4.2, A4.6
  Clinical Trial Products A13.5
Crude Plant (Vegetable Drug) A7, Gls.
Cryogenic Vessels Gls.
  Checks Before Filling A6.17
  Filling A6.26–A6.27
Cryoprecipitation of blood fractions A14.20
Culture Media 6.20, A2.34
Cylinders A6.9, Gls.
  Filling A6.7–A6.8, A6.19–A6.25
  Labelling A6.29
  Preparation for Filling A6.16–A6.18
  Segregation A6.4
  Storage A6.31–A6.32

Decontamination 5.19, A2.5, A2.15, A5.5, A5.47
Dedicated areas 3.6
Blood Products A14.6
Destruction of Clinical Trial Returns A13.45 – A13.47
Disinfectants A1.32–A1.33
Disinfection A5.16, A5.32, A5.51
Distribution:
  Radiopharmaceuticals A3.10
  Records 4.25, 8.12
Documentation Ch. 4
  Biological Medicinal Products A2.23–A2.24
  Clinical Trial Products A13.8 – A13.10

Contained/Clean Areas A5. 20
General 4.1–4.9
Herbal Products A7.5–A7.6
Quality Control 6.7–6.10
Radiation Treatment A12.42–A12.45
Required 4.10–4.29
Donation of blood A14.1 – A14.11
Dose Mapping A12.10
Electron Beam Irradiation A12.25–A12.26
Gamma Irradiation A12.17–A12.22
Dosimetry:
Radiation Sterilisation A1.63
Radiation Treatment A12.4–A12.8, A12.10
Drains 3.11, A1.21
Dust 3.14, 5.11, A4.1, A7.4

Ectoparasiticides A4.5–A4.6
Effluents A2.19, A5.11, A5.32, A5.52
Electron Beam Irradiation A12
Design A12.23–A12.24
Dose Mapping A12.25–A12.26
Processing A12.40–A12.41
Electronic Data Processing Systems 4.9, A11
Emulsions, Sterile A1.5, A1.6
Endotoxins, Monitoring for A1.85
Equipment 3.34–3.44
Biological Products A2.6–A2.20
Blood products A14.6
Chromatography A2.40
Clinical Trial Products A13.5 – A13.7
Contained/Clean Areas A5.11–A5.12, A5.17, A5.21–A5.27
Liquids, Creams & Ointments A9.1–A9.3
Log Books 4.28–4.29
Maintenance 3.35, A1.29–A1.30, A5.26
Medicinal Gases A6.2–A6.10
Operating Procedures 4.27
Pressurized Aerosols for Inhalation A10.2–A10.3
Radiopharmaceuticals A3.2–A3.5
Sterile Products A1.27–A1.31
Ethylene Oxide Sterilisation A1.67–A1.73
Exotic Organisms Gls.
Experimental Products A13

Feedingstuffs, Medicated A4.1–A4.4

Fermenters A2.35, A5.50
Filling:
  Cryogenic Vessels A6.26–A6.27
  Gas Cylinders A6.7–A6.8, A6.19–A6.25
  Pressurized Aerosols for Inhalation A10.1, A10.7–A10.8
Filling Processes:
  Immunological Veterinary Products A5.60–A5.63
  Liquids, Creams & Ointments A9.8
Filtration:
  Air A1.1, A1.24, A5.11
  Fluids for Pressurized Aerosols A10.5
  Medicinal Products A1.47, A1.74–A1.79
Finished Products 5.58–5.60, Gls.
  Assessment 6.3
  Quarantine 5.5, 5.58
  Release 4.24, A6.30, A11.19
  Retention of Samples 6.14
  Specifications 4.13
Food & Drink 2.17
Fractionation of blood A14.11 – A14.25
Freeze Driers A5.27

Gamma Irradiation A12
  Design A12.14–A12.16
  Dose Mapping A12.17–A12.22
  Processing A12.35–A12.39
Garments, See Clothing
Gases, Medicinal A6
  Labelling A6.29
  Liquefied A6.10, A6.12, A6.26
  Personnel A6.1
  Premises & Equipment A6.2–A6.10
  Production & Quality Control A6.11–A6.28
  Storage/Release A6.30–A6.32
Good Manufacturing Practice (GMP) 1.3
Good Manufacturing Practice for Investigational Products A13

Hand-washing Facilities 2.19, A1.22
Heat Sterilisation A1.55–A1.61
Herbal Products A7, Gls.
  Documentation A7.5–A7.6
  Premises A7.1–A7.4
  Quality Control A7.8–A7.9
  Sampling A7.7

Hydrostatic Test A6.17
Hygiene 2.13–2.20, A1.10

Immunological Veterinary Products A5
Animals & Animal Houses A5.28–A5.31
Disinfection/Waste Disposal A5.32
Equipment A5.21–A5.27
Personnel A5.1–A5.5, A5.45
Premises A5.6–A5.20
Production A5.33–A5.64
Quality Control A5.35–A5.36, A5.65–A5.68
Imported Products 2.4
In-process Controls 3.17, 6.18, Gls.
Biological Medicinal Products A2.41
Immunological Veterinary Products A5.65
Inactivated Products A5.57–A5.58
Incubators A5.25, A5.55
Infected Gls.
Infectious Diseases 2.15, A2.3
Infusion Solutions A1.47, A1.85
Inhalation, Pressurized Aerosol Products for A10
Inspection:
Parenteral Products A1.82
Self Ch. 9
Intermediate Products Gls.
Biological Medicinal Products A2.42
Immunological Veterinary Products A5.66
Processing Operations 5.35–5.39
Receipt 5.6
Specifications 4.12, A2.24
Investigational Medicinal Products, GMP for A13
Investigator A13 Gls
Irradiation, See Radiation Treatment

Key Personnel 2.3–2.7

Labelling 5.12–5.13, 5.49–5.53
Clinical Trial Products A13.18
Gas Cylinders A6.29
Pipework 3.42
Sample Containers 6.13
Starting Materials 5.29
Sterile Products A1.54
Laminar Air Flow Systems A1.3

Leakage Tests A6.25, A10.9
Lighting, Production Areas 3.16
Liquefiable Gases Gls.
Liquefied Medicinal Gases A6.10, A6.12, A6.26
Liquids A9
  Premises & Equipment A9.1–A9.3
  Production A9.4–A9.9
Log Books, Equipment 4.28–4.29
Lot, See Batch

Maintenance:
  Equipment 3.35, A1.29–A1.30, A5.26
  Premises 3.2
  Workshops 3.32
Manifolds A6.5, A6.14, A6.20, Gls.
Manufacture Gls.
Manufacturer Gls.
Manufacturing Formulae 4.1, 4.14
  Clinical Trial Products A13.14
Media:
  Immunological Veterinary Products A5.38–A5.39
  Sterilisation A2.37, A5.39
Medical Examinations 2.14, A5.3
Medicated Feedingstuffs A4.1–A4.4
Medicinal Gases, See Gases, Medicinal
Medicinal Plants A7, Gls.
Medicinal Products Gls.
Microbial Cultures A2
Microbiological Monitoring:
  Clean Areas A1.32–A1.35
  Radiation Treatment A12.46
Monoclonal Antibodies A2, A2.11

Ointments A9
  Premises & Equipment A9.1–A9.3
  Production A9.4–A9.9
  Sterile A1.5, A1.6
One-shot Filling Process A10.1

Packaging Gls.
  Batch Records 4.18
  Clinical Trial Products A13.15 – A13.19, A13.26
  Instructions 4.1, 4.16
  Operations 5.44–5.57

Premises 3.15
Packaging Materials S.40–S.43, Gls.
Printed 5.41, 5.50–5.53
Sampling A8
Specifications 4.11
Storage 3.25, 5.41
Parenteral Products/Solutions A1.5, A1.6, A1.82
Penicillins, Veterinary Products Containing A4.7
Personnel Ch. 2
Authorized, Data Entry/Amendment A11.8, A11.10
Biological Medicinal Products A2.1–A2.5, A2.32
Clean Areas A1.7–A1.16, A1.41
Clinical Trial Products A13.4
Computerized Systems A11.1
General 2.1
Hygiene 2.13–2.20, A1.10
Immunological Veterinary Products A5.1–A5.5, A5.45
Key 2.3–2.7
Medicinal Gases A6.1
Principle Ch. 2
Radiopharmaceuticals A3.1
Restricted Access 2.11, 3.5, 5.16, A5.19
Sampling A8.1
Training, See Training, Personnel
Pest Control A4.1
Pipes/Pipelines A1. 20, A2.17
Connections 5.14, A6.5
Labelling 3.42
Water 3.43
Plants, Medicinal A7, Gls.
Plasma A14
Premises for posting A14.17
Premises Ch. 3
Biological Medicinal Products A2.6–A2.20
Blood collection A14.5 – A14.6
Clinical Trial Products A13.5 – A13.7
General 3.1–3.5
Herbal Products A7.1–A7.4
Immunological Veterinary Products A5.6–A5.20
Liquids, Creams & Ointments A9.1–A9.3
Medicinal Gases A6.2–A6.10
Pressurized Aerosols for Inhalation A10.2–A10.3
Radiation Treatment A12.28
Radiopharmaceuticals A3.2–A3.5

Sterile Products A1.17–A1.26
Veterinary Medicinal Products A4.1
Premixes for Medicated Feedingstuffs A4.1–A4.4
Pressurized Aerosol Products for Inhalation A10
Printed Packaging Materials 5.41, 5.50–5.53
Procedures 4.1, 4.19–4.29, Gls.
Complaints 8.2
Deviations from 5.15
Recalls 8.9
Processing Instructions 4.1, 4.14–4.15
Herbal Products A7.6
Processing Operations 5.35–5.39
Biological Products A2.10–A2.14, A2.34–A2.40
Blood and Plasma Products A14.7 – A14.25
Immunological Veterinary Products A5.46–A5.64
Radiation Treatment A12.29–A12.41
Sterile Products A1.36–A1.49
Production Ch. 5, Gls.
Areas 3.6–3.17, 6.4
Biological Medicinal Products A2.25–A2.40
Clinical Trial Products A13.20 – A13.29
Duties of Head of Department 2.5, 2.7
General 5.1–5.17
Herbal Products A7.4
Immunological Veterinary Products A5.33–A5.64
Liquids, Creams & Ointments A9.4–A9.9
Medicinal Gases A6.11–A6.28
Pressurized Aerosols for Inhalation A10.4–A10.9
Prevention of Cross-contamination 3.6, 5.18–5.20
Radiopharmaceuticals A3.6–A3.7
Validation 5.21–3.24, A1.38, A1.49, A2.38, A5.59

Qualification Gls.
Qualified Person:
Complaints 8.1
Contract Manufacture & 7.11
Duties 2.4, A3.8
Medicinal Gases A6.1
Recalls 8.8
Release of Finished Product 4.24, A11.19
Quality Assurance 1.2, 2.12
Clinical Trial Products A13.2
Quality Control Ch. 6
Areas (Laboratories) 3.26–3.29

Basic Requirements 1.4
Biological Medicinal Products A2.41–A2.44
Blood Products A14.1 – A14.4, A14.12 - A14.19
Clinical Trial Products A13.30 – A13.33
Complaints & 8.3
Definition 1.4
Documentation 6.7–6.10
Duties of Head of Department 2.6, 2.7
General 6.l–6.4
Good Laboratory Practice 6.S–6.22
Herbal Products A7.8–A7.9
Immunological Veterinary Products A5.35–A5.36, A5.65–A5.68
Medicinal Gases A6.11–A6.28
Pressurized Aerosols for Inhalation A10.4–A10.9
Radiopharmaceuticals A3.8–A3.9
Sampling 6.11–6.14
Sterile Products A1.83–A1.85
Testing 6.15–6.22, A2.21
Quality Management Ch.1
Clinical Trial Products A13.1
Quarantine 3.21, 5.5, Gls.
Finished Products 5.5, 5.58
Medicinal Gases A6.30

Radiation Indicators A1.63, A12.31
Radiation Sterilisation A1.62–A1.66
Radiation Treatment A12
Commissioning of the Plant A12.12–A12.27
Documentation A12.42–A12.45
Dosimetry A12.4–A12.8
Microbiological Monitoring A12.46
Premises A12.28
Process Validation A12.9–A12.11
Processing A12.29–A12.41
Responsibilities A12.1–A12.3
Radiopharmaceuticals A3, Gls.
Distribution & Recalls A3.10
Personnel A3.1
Premises & Equipment A3.2–A3.5
Production A3.6–A3.7
Quality Control A3.8–A3.9
Re-Commissioning, Radiation Treatment Plant A12.27
Reagents, Laboratory 6.19–6.21
Recalled Products 3.23, 8.8–8.15, A3.10, A13.36

Receipts:
Incoming Materials 5.3, 5.5–5.6
Procedures & Records 4.19–4.21
Recombinant DNA Technology, Products of A2, A2.11
Reconciliations 5.8, 5.56, 8.14, A5.64, A12.42, Gls.
Records 4.1, 4.19–4.29
Batch, See Batch Records
Clinical Trial Products A13.8 – A13.10
Complaints 8.5–8.6
Contract Manufacture 7.13
Distribution 4.25, 8.12, A13.42
Quality Control Tests 6.17
Self Inspections 9.3
Recovery 5.61–5.65, Gls.
Reference Samples – see Samples, reference
Refreshment Rooms 3.30
Rejected Materials 3.23, 5.61–5.65
Procedures 4.24
Reprocessing 5.62–5.64
Release of Finished Products 4.24, A6.30, A11.19, A13.31, A13.39
Reprocessing 5.62–5.64, Gls.
Rest Rooms 3.30
Retention Samples, See Samples, reference
Returns 3.23, 5.61–5.65, A13.34 - A13.44, Gls.

Samples, Reference 6.12
Biological Medicinal Products A2.41
Blood Products A14.26
Immunological Veterinary Products A5.66
Radiopharmaceuticals A3.9
Retention 6.14, A4.8–A4.9, A5.66, A13.29
Storage 3.27
Veterinary Medicinal Products A4.8–A4.9
Sampling:
Biological Products A2.35
Herbal Products A7.7
Medicinal Gases A6.13
Packaging Materials A8
Personnel A8.1
Procedures & Records 4.22
Quality Control 6.11–6.14
Starting Materials 3.22, A8
Sterile Products A1. 84
Sanitation, Clean Areas A1.32–A1.25

Security, Electronic Data A11.13
Seed Lots A2.27–A2.33, A5.40–A5.45, Gls.
Self Inspection Ch. 9
Sinks A1. 21
Smoking 2.17
Software, Computerized Systems A11.5
Specifications 4.1, 4.10–4.13
  Biological Medicinal Products A2.23–A2.24
  Clinical Trial Products A13.12
  Irradiation Process A12.11
  Starting Materials 4.11, A2.23, A5.34, A7.5
Spillages, Accidental A5. 47
Sponsor of Clinical Trial A13 Gls
Starting Materials 5.25–5.34, Gls.
  Biological Medicinal Products A2.25–A2.26
  Blood Products A14.2 – A14.16
  Clinical Trial Products A13.20 – A13.21
  Delivery 5.27–5.28
  Dispensing 5.32–5.34
  Herbal Products A7.5
  Identity Testing A8.2–A8.3
  Immunological Veterinary Products A5.34–A5.37
  Labelling 5.29
  Purchase 5.25–5.26
  Retention of Samples 6.14
  Sampling 3.22, A8
  Specifications 4.11, A2.23, A5.34, A7.5
  Sterile Products A1. 42
  Sterilisation A2.26, A5.37
  Weighing 3.13
Steam Sterilisation A1.58–A1.60
Sterile Products A1, A3.4, A4.10
  Aseptic Preparations A1.6
  Finishing A1.80–A1.82
  General A1.1–A1.6
  Processing A1.36–A1.49
  Quality Control A1.83–A1.85
  Terminally Sterilised A1.5
  See also Clean Areas
Sterilisation A1.50–A1.79
  Clinical Trial Products A13.7
  Dry Heat A1. 61
  Equipment A1.28, A2.17, A5.24, A5.27
  Ethylene Oxide A1.67–A1.73

Filtration A1.74–A1.79
Heat A1.55–A1.61
Media A2.37, A5.39
Radiation A1.62–A1.66
Starting Materials A2.26, A5.37
Steam A1.58–A1.60
Sterility Gls.
Sterility Test A1.83
Storage 5.7
Areas 3.18–3.25
Herbal Products A7.1–A7.3
Immunological Veterinary Products A5.25, A5.63
Liquids, Creams & Ointments A9.9
Medicinal Gases A6.30–A6.32
Packaging Materials 3.25, 5.41
Recalled Products 8.13
Rejected Materials 5.61
Seed Lots & Cell Banks A2.31–A2.33, A5.44–A5.45
Starting Materials 5.29
Sterile Products A1. 73
Suspensions, Sterile A1.5, A1.6
System Gls.

Testing:
Procedures & Records 4.23
Quality Control 6.15–6.22, A2.21
Toilet Facilities 3.31
Training, Personnel 2.8–2.12, A1.8, A2.1, A3.1, A5.1–A5.2, A8.1
Transfer Operations:
Contained/Clean Areas A5.48–A5.54
Liquids, Creams & Ointments A9.5–A9.6
Medicinal Gases A6.12–A6.13
Tuberculin Products A2.4, A2.8
Two-shot Filling Process A10.1, A10.8

Vaccinations A2.3, A5.3
Vaccines A2.12, A2.21
Validation Gls.
Clinical Trial Products A13.7, A13.22 – A13.24
Computerized Systems A11.2
Production Processes 5.21–5.24, A1.38, A1.49, A2.38, A5.59
Radiation Treatment A12.9–A12.11
Sampling Starting Materials A8.2–A8.3
Sterilisation A1.50, A1.64, A1.67, A1.77

Valves:
Cleaning A2.17
Metering, for Aerosols A10.4, A10.6
Ventilation, See Air Supply Systems
Veterinary Products A4
Ectoparasiticides A4.5–A4.6
Immunological, See Immunological Veterinary Products
Penicillin Containing A4.7
Premixes for Medicated Feedingstuffs A4.1–A4.4
Retention of Samples A4.8–A4.9
Sterile A4.10
Vials, Capping A5.62
Viral Inactivation of Blood Products A14.18 – A14.25
Visitors 2.11, A2.3

Warning Systems A1.26
Washing Facilities 3.31, A1.22
Waste Disposal A2.19, A5.11, A5.32, A5.52
Water:
Monitoring A1.40, A1.85
Pipes 3.43
Treatment A1.31, A1.40, A9.4
Weighing Rooms, Starting Materials 3.13
Whole blood processing A14, A14.27 – A14.29
Workshops, Maintenance 3.32

Yields, Checks on 5.8, A5.64

Part Five

Defective medicines report centre

5. MEDICINES CONTROL AGENCY: DEFECTIVE MEDICINES REPORT CENTRE

Manufacturers and importers are obliged to report to the licensing authority any quality defect in a medicinal product which could result in a recall or restriction on supply. Other users and distributors of medicinal products are encouraged to do this. The Medicines Control Agency operates a round-the-clock Defective Medicines Report Centre (DMRC) to receive reports on products for human use and to co-ordinate the necessary assessment and action. (The Veterinary Medicines Directorate operates a comparable system in relation to veterinary medicinal products and the Medical Devices Directorate a system dealing with medical devices.)

Telephone Numbers

Office Hours (08.30 – 17.45)	**071 273 0574**
Silent Hours	**071 210 5368/5371**
Fax (manned in office hours only)	**071 273 0676**

Address:

Defective Medicines Report Centre,
Medicines Control Agency,
Room 1801, Market Towers
1 Nine Elms Lane
London SW8 5NQ

Aim

To minimise the hazard to patients arising from the distribution of defective medicinal products for human use by providing an emergency assessment and communications system between the suppliers (manufacturer and distributors), the regulatory authorities and the users.

Scope

Defective medicinal products for human use:

– one whose quality does not conform to the requirements of its product licence or in some other way is not of the quality intended.

The DMRC does not deal with:

– adverse drug reactions	(Refer to ADR Business of MCA)	Dial 100 and ask for "CSM Freephone" or telephone 071 273 0400
– defective medical devices	(Refer to Medical Devices Directorate of DH)	Tel: 071 636 6811
– defective veterinary medicinal products	(Refer to Veterinary Medicines Directorate of MAFF)	Tel: 0932 336911

Details to be Reported

The report of a suspected defective product should contain, as far as possible:

Product name, manufacturer, supplier, batch/lot number, PL number, dosage form, strength, container type/size, expiry date, name and position of person reporting and where contact(s) for further information can be made, and a summary of the suspected defect.

When the report is made by the licence holder, the following additional information is likely to be required at the same time as the report is made or soon after:

Site of manufacture, date when first distributed, distribution pattern, any remaining stock (including any returns).

Action by DMRC

The defect report is assessed professionally and the necessary action is discussed and agreed with the responsible licence holder. In some cases, where the defect presents a significant hazard to health, it may be necessary for MCA to issue a 'Drug Alert' letter to UK Health Authorities and a 'Rapid Alert' letter to EC and overseas authorities as appropriate, notifying a 'caution in use', quarantine or recall by the manufacturer of the defective batch. Appropriate advisory classification of urgency is included in the Drug Alert letters:

Class 1	Immediate action including out of hours
Class 2	Action within 48 hours
Class 3	Action within 5 days
Class 4	Caution in use

Printed in the United Kingdom for HMSO.
Dd.0296437, 11/93, C100, 3396/4, 5673, 259650.